SURGERY
A layman's guide to common operations

Edward L. Stern, M.D.

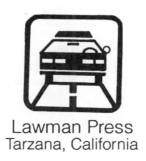

Lawman Press
Tarzana, California

To my grandchildren
Veronica, Erica and Shane

Special thanks
to my wife, Bette,
my son Ronald and
my daughter-in-law Nancy.
Without their encouragement and and help this
book would not have been written.

Published by
Lawman Press
18653 Ventura Blvd., Suite 314-B
Tarzana, CA 91356 U.S.A.

First printing 1989
10 9 8 7 6 5 4 3 2 1

ILLUSTRATIONS AND COVER DESIGN BY NANCY STERN
DESIGN BY WORDS & DEEDS, INC., LOS ANGELES

Printed in the United States of America

Library of Congress Catalog Card Number 88-081920
ISBN 0-944711-01-4

CONTENTS

DISCLAIMER

This book is designed to provide information in regard to the subject matter covered. It is sold with the understanding that the publisher and author are not engaged in rendering legal, medical or other professional services. Further, the function of this book is to explain medical procedures and techniques. It should not be used as a means of self-diagnosis or treatment. If medical assistance is required, the services of a competent physician or other health care professional should be sought.

It is not the purpose of this book to reprint all information that is otherwise available to the author and/or publisher but to complement, amplify and supplement other texts.

Effort has been made to make this guide as complete and accurate as possible. However, there may be mistakes both typographical and in content. Therefore, this text should only be used as a general guide and not as the ultimate source of medical information. Furthermore, this guide contains information only up to the printing date.

The purpose of this book is to educate and entertain. The author and Lawman Press shall have neither liability nor responsibility to any person or entity with respect to any loss or damage caused or alleged to be caused directly or indirectly by the information contained in this publication.

PREFACE

I recognized the need for a book covering this subject matter more than twenty years ago when I left general practice and entered an anesthesiology residency. I discovered in my pre-anesthetic visits with patients that many of them had no idea what was going to be done in surgery and what, if any, would be the long-lasting effects. They would ask: "Where will my incision be located?" "Will it leave a scar?" "How can I digest my food after my gallbladder is removed?" "Will I still menstruate after my hysterectomy?" They simply had no idea what organs or tissues were going to be removed during surgery. If you understand what surgery consists of, it helps you to better understand the postoperative course. As I continue in my career as an anesthesiologist, my opinion as to the need for a book like this is continually reinforced.

Facts about common surgeries and how they are performed are explained in understandable, nontechnical terms. Whenever a medical term is used, its definition is included. It would be very difficult in a book of this sort to differentiate between the sexes when talking about general medical conditions, so I have chosen to refer to the patient in the male gender when discussing a condition that may affect both men and women. For convenience I also use the male pronoun to refer to the surgeon; in reality, of course, a doctor may be a man or a woman.

Chapter one is an explanation of anesthesia and surgical monitoring. I hope you will take the time to read this chapter as it corrects many of the misconceptions surrounding anesthesia and I believe it will be of interest.

This book is not a medical treatment guide; diagnosis or treatment of medical problems should be based on recommendations by your doctor. Use the book as an explanatory guide to better understand medical discussions between you and your doctor. Due to limited space and the book's intended use, many facts, treatments, complications and descriptions are not mentioned at all or are not fully covered. Also, I have simplified many surgical procedures and the medical facts relating to them.

Because some of the objectives of this book are to make it interesting and understandable to the layman (the average reader would probably not find a discussion of the sodium and potassium ions in the intracellular and interstitial fluids interesting or understandable), in-depth discussion of complicated matters has been omitted.

ANESTHESIA AND MONITORING

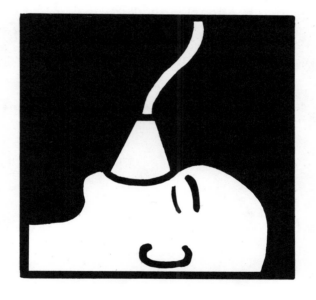

In general, it is a good policy to use the least possible amount of anesthesia that allows the surgeon to perform the surgery and the patient to be comfortable.

ANESTHESIA

Frequently in my practice of anesthesia, patients tell me they are more afraid of the anesthetic than the surgery. Concerns about the risks of anesthesia and surgery are, of course, legitimate. Although anesthesia is very safe, there are some patients who do not awaken. Does this mean that you should forgo needed surgery because of the fear of anesthesia? I don't think so. We all take calculated risks everyday of our lives, usually without giving them a second thought. Surgeons now perform far more complex surgeries on more seriously ill patients than ever before, and surgery is now safer than it ever has been. The reasons for this are multifaceted and complex, and start with improvements in training of all medical personnel—not only the surgeon and anesthesiologist, but also the nursing staff. They cannot be given all the credit, however. Some very significant anesthesia monitoring equipment developed during the last few years has also made its contribution.

How Anesthesia Works

Many people are under the misconception that general anesthesia (where the patient is asleep during surgery) consists of nothing more than receiving a preoperative shot and an injection of sodium pentothal in the operating room, with the anesthesiologist then free to leave. This is as far from the

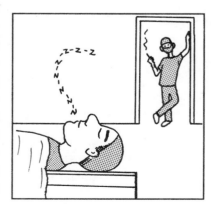

truth as the idea that surgery is finished as soon as the surgeon makes the skin incision. In both cases this is only the beginning. Let's look at some of the interesting and mostly unknown functions performed by the anesthesiologist.

The anesthetic drugs depress normal lung function, making it necessary for the anesthesiologist to continually breathe for the patient. Without this support of respiration, breathing would be greatly reduced or entirely stopped. (This is one of the reasons I chuckle when patients ask if I am going to stay for the whole operation.) There are many unwanted or exaggerated side effects of anesthetic drugs; if their level is not constantly adjusted, they can cause considerable harm or even death. Besides their adverse effects on the lungs, anesthetic agents decrease the functions of the heart and blood vessels. This causes a lowering of the blood pressure and reduced profusion of blood to the vital organs.

We also administer muscle-relaxing drugs that completely paralyze all voluntary muscles of the body. (Breathing is one of these voluntary muscle functions, as you can control its rate and depth.) One such commonly used drug, curare, is related to the poison used by South American Indians on the tips of their hunting arrows. Once struck, their prey falls to the ground, apparently dead. Actually it is only paralyzed— unable to move, make any sound, or breathe, and will subsequently die of asphyxiation.

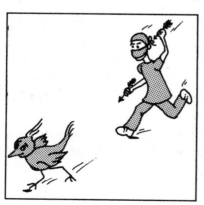

One reason we use these drugs is that even when the patient is asleep under anesthesia there is a certain degree of tension in all muscles. This tone is especially strong in the muscles surrounding the abdomen and exerts enough pressure to interfere with abdominal surgery by pushing the intestines into the surgical site. The unwanted bowel obstructs the surgeon's view, making it difficult, if not impos-

> The anesthetic drugs depress normal lung function, making it necessary for the anesthesiologist to continually breathe for the patient.

sible, to perform the surgery. Using muscle-relaxing drugs keeps the surgical area free of the clutter of unwanted intestines.

Another common use of these drugs is to facilitate the passage of a breathing tube through the mouth down into the trachea (windpipe). During many surgeries the face is not accessible to the anesthesiologist, making it impossible to put a mask on the patient's face and breathe for him. And during abdominal surgery the surgical site is packed with cloth sponges which exert pressure on the diaphragm which then compresses the lungs. This decreases the ability of the anesthesiologist to adequately breathe for the patient. The solution to these problems is the passage of an endotracheal tube into the trachea where it acts as an air conduit to breathe for the patient. This is a hollow tube of good-sized diameter and must be inserted under direct vision. First we use medication to relax the patient's jaw and vocal cord muscles. Next we insert an instrument with a light on the end of a metal blade into the patient's mouth. This illuminates the paralyzed vocal cords while the endotracheal tube is inserted between them into the trachea.

We always tell our patients not to eat or drink anything after midnight the night before surgery. This is not, as most people think, because they will become nauseated and vomit after surgery. Rather it is because of a little flap of tissue, the epiglottis, that closes the opening of the windpipe when we swallow. This prevents food from passing down through the windpipe and entering the lungs. Under anesthesia the epiglottis loses its ability to do this protective maneuver, leaving the lungs vulnerable to the intrusion of stomach contents.

There are many reasons why pressure builds up in and around the stomach while the patient is anesthetized. This pressure could cause anything present in the stomach to regurgitate into the throat and run down into the trachea and lungs. If solid food is regurgitated, it could produce complete obstruction of the airway. Or acidic stomach fluid could enter and irritate the lungs, causing pneumonia. Needless to say, these are serious complications. To prevent this occurrence there is a balloon on the end of the endotracheal tube that can be inflated, blocking anything solid or liquid from entering the trachea.

TYPES OF ANESTHESIA

The different types of anesthesia range from the patient being completely asleep to just being numbed in a small, local area. In general, it is a good policy to use the least possible amount of anesthesia that allows the surgeon to perform the surgery and the patient to be comfortable. There are, of course, overriding factors that will also influence this decision. If the area to be operated on is infected, it might not be prudent to insert a needle and possibly spread the infection. When patients are fearful, or have a low pain threshold, general anesthesia might be the better choice.

Local Anesthesia

With a local anesthetic, the local anesthetic solution is injected around the surgical site, making it insensitive to pain. With the popularity of outpatient surgery, local anesthetics have become the primary anesthetic in some major cases, such as an inguinal hernia repair (see Hernia Repair, p. 111). There are many types of local anesthetic solutions. Some have a very short duration, as little as thirty minutes; others can last up to six hours. The type of local anesthetic used varies with the needs of the surgery. There is no free lunch: As safe as local anesthetics are, severe reactions to them can occur.

Regional Anesthesia

This type of anesthesia numbs a specific part of the body—from the waist down, for example. This is accomplished with a spinal or epidural anesthetic. The well-known saddle block, for many years the anesthetic of choice for delivering babies, is actually a spinal anesthetic. It is called a saddle block because it numbs the same area that touches a saddle while horseback riding.

In a spinal anesthetic a long, thin needle is inserted through the skin of the lower back and then between the vertebrae (spinal bones) into the fluid of the spinal canal. A small amount of local anesthetic is injected into the spinal fluid where it blocks nerve impulses. Any painful stimuli originating below this area won't be felt, as it can't be communicated past this block to the brain. If the concentration of the anesthetic drug is strong enough, all the corresponding muscles will be paralyzed.

In contrast, with an epidural anesthetic a much larger needle is inserted in the same manner as a spinal except that it is stopped just before it reaches the thin layer of tissue that covers the spinal canal. Instead of injecting a small volume of local anesthetic into the spinal fluid, a large volume is placed outside of the spinal canal to numb the nerves that fan out after leaving the spinal canal. The individual nerves leave at different levels to innervate their appropriate end organs. Because this is such a large area to cover, compared to the spinal, a much larger volume must be used. The anesthesiologist can also render an extremity such as an arm or leg numb by injecting the nerves supplying it with a local anesthetic. This technique is frequently used for hand or foot surgery.

General Anesthesia

Usually some type of premedication is given to the patient, either an hour before surgery in the patient's room or just minutes before surgery in the operating room. In the operating room medication is given by the intravenous route which takes effect rapidly as it does not have to be absorbed from the tissues. This injection usually contains a drying agent and a strong narcotic. The drying agent reduces saliva or other fluids in the upper respiratory tract. The narcotic reduces apprehension and creates some sedation and euphoria. This reduces the effects of circulating adrenaline that the anxiety of the surgery has produced. Adrenaline can produce undesirable side effects under anesthesia, such as high blood pressure and irregular heart beats.

More than once I have heard it said: He choked because he swallowed his tongue. You can't swallow your tongue, but under anesthesia the muscles around the throat relax, causing the tongue to fall back and obstruct the airway. In

> You can't swallow your tongue, but under anesthesia the muscles around the throat relax, causing the tongue to fall back and obstruct the airway.

anesthesia we use an oral airway to combat this problem. This is a firm rubber device, about three inches long, which curves slightly to fit into the throat. It is inserted after the patient is asleep to keep the tongue in a more forward position. The oral airway, endotracheal tube and anesthetic gases are irritating to the mucous membranes of the respiratory tract. The body's natural defense is to secrete protective fluids. The second part of the premedication injection, the drying agent, counteracts this response. It is the combined effect of the drying agent and withholding fluids for many hours before surgery that causes the dry mouth experienced before and after surgery.

Next, all the anesthetic monitors are attached to the patient and an intravenous line is started in one of the upper extremities to allow replacement of fluids that are lost and to provide a direct route into the blood stream for injection of medications. When injected intravenously they exert their effects far faster than when injected into a muscle. Sodium pentothal is now injected into the intravenous line and with minimal or no sensation the patient becomes unconscious. People are often surprised when I tell them that after they are asleep I am going to keep them asleep with gas. Sodium pentothal is a wonderful drug with which to go to sleep, but it has very few analgesic (pain relieving) properties. The anesthetic gases, on the other hand, have the high analgesic

> Sodium pentothal is a wonderful drug with which to go to sleep, but it has very few pain relieving properties.

effect necessary to keep the patient from feeling pain and moving. And because of their high degree of potency, the depth of anesthesia can be quickly changed. These factors make gases more suitable anesthetic agents.

MONITORS

Anesthetic agents, as with many good things, can have serious and undesirable side effects. They can reduce respirations, heart rate and blood pressure. Some predisposed patients can develop a malignant and frequently fatal rise in body temperature. In others, fatal amounts of electrolytes (such as potassium) can be released into the blood stream, causing the heart to stop beating. Anesthetics can also cause strokes, heart attacks, cardiac or respiratory arrest, as well as kidney or liver failure. As surgeries have become more complex, so has the practice of anesthesia. It is now necessary to know a great deal more about the patient's condition. These few examples of complications are not given to frighten the reader, but only to better help him understand why monitoring has become so important in the practice of anesthesia.

Oxygen Saturation Monitor

This is our newest and probably best monitor for detecting problems early—frequently while they are still clinically undetectable. Lack of adequate oxygen is the most feared and devastating complication of anesthesia. It is not just the brain which cannot tolerate oxygen deprivation, but other vital organs as well. Until now, we had to rely on the late signs of cyanosis (bluish discoloration of the skin) or the slowing of the heart from lack of fuel (oxygen) to contract its muscles. The probe of the oxygen saturation monitor fits over the tip of a finger where it emits an infrared signal which the machine converts into an oxygen saturation value. It gives a continual reading of the percent by which the blood is saturated with oxygen.

Carbon Dioxide Monitor

This monitor connects to the hoses that bring the anesthetic gases to and from the patient. The carbon dioxide measurement at the end of each breath is the same as that in the blood, so we are in reality measuring the concentration in the blood. Carbon dioxide is a waste product of living cells and is produced through cell metabolism and eliminated in part by the lungs. These values are helpful in evaluating the adequacy of respirations and the early diagnoses of other complications of anesthesia.

Temperature Monitor

As mentioned earlier, one of the complications of anesthesia is a sudden and lethal rise in body temperature. This fever is so severe that submerging the patient in ice and infusing cold intravenous solutions will not abate the high temperature. Even inserting tubes into body orifices and flushing them with ice water is of little help. Luckily, we now have a specific medication that, if given early, can help bring this condition under control. In children there is the problem of intravenous solutions at room temperature which, if you have ever had surgery, you know is well below the body's 98.6 degrees. These factors cause the opposite effect — lowering of the body's temperature. Early warning in the rising or lowering of body temperature is important in averting major complications. We have thermometers that attach to the skin giving us a continuous temperature reading, making it easy to note trends up or down.

Muscle Stimulators

The muscle-relaxing (actually paralyzing) drugs come in short- or long-acting forms. There is no way to lessen the effects of the short-acting muscle relaxants, but the effects of the long-acting ones can be reversed. This is only possible if paralysis is not complete. With the muscle stimulator, electrical probes are placed over specific nerves. An electrical charge is then administered through the skin to that nerve. The muscles activated by this nerve will contract in accordance to the degree that they are not paralyzed. That is, the more paralyzed they are, the less they will respond to the stimuli. It is normal practice to attempt to keep the muscles

> Patients have told me they have
> heard that anesthesia places
> a patient close to death.

less than 100 percent paralyzed. This helps to ensure that the shorter-acting drugs will soon wear off, and the long-acting ones can be reversed. By judging the degree of muscle twitch the level of paralysis can be estimated.

Precordial Stethoscope

Listening to breath sounds is another method of determining whether or not there is adequate exchange of gases into and out of the lungs. This is similar to your family doctor listening to your chest. Listening to the quality, rate and rhythm of the heart beat is also helpful. By the judicious placing of a stethoscope on the patient's chest, the anesthesiologist can hear both the lungs and the heart.

Electrocardiograph

Your internist is not the only one to gain valuable information from the electrical impulses given off by the heart. The electrocardiogram (EKG) done in the doctor's office gives the doctor information about the condition of the heart at that moment. Since the patient's condition is not likely to change quickly, this is usually adequate. In anesthesia, however, the condition of the patient is changing from moment to moment. Therefore, the EKG that we use is displayed on a television monitor and constantly updated during surgery.

Automatic Blood Pressure Monitor

Blood pressure measurements are one of the oldest and most important monitors in anesthesia. Patients have told me they have heard that anesthesia places a patient close to death. It is true that it renders him unconscious, limiting his ability to maintain normal blood pressure, heart rate and respirations. It is mandatory that the blood pressure be maintained at levels high enough to profuse the vital organs of the body. This monitor automatically checks the patient's blood pressure at time intervals set by the anesthesiologist.

Disconnect Alarms

It is a common practice to place a patient on a mechanical ventilator during long surgeries. This machine automatically pushes the gases into the lungs and allows the expelled gases to be removed. If the ventilator should inadvertently become disconnected from the patient, breathing would be interrupted and, if not detected quickly, death would occur. With a disconnect alarm in use during such an occurrence, the anesthesiologist is alerted immediately by the alarm beep.

Using so many monitors with disconnect alarms can get confusing. When the anesthesiologist does hear an alarm, it's not always easy to determine which monitor it is coming from. On several occasions in my own experience, the beep I have searched so hard to find has turned out to come not from one of my alarms, but rather the surgeon's pager!

I hope this brief discussion of monitors has helped make it clearer to the reader some of the reasons anesthesia is safer today. When I started my practice of anesthesia twenty-five years ago, the only monitors I had were my precordial stethoscope and a hand-inflated blood pressure cuff. You may have noticed that nowhere was there mention of a monitor that would tell the "depth" of anesthesia. This is a value judgment, governed by the collective readings of all monitors, plus the experience of the anesthesiologist.

HEMORRHOIDECTOMY

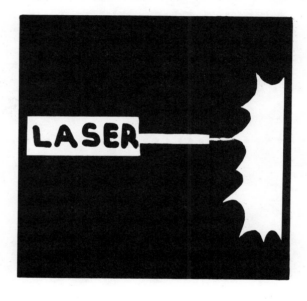

Hemorrhoids are usually painless—
the complications of hemorrhoids
cause the discomfort.

Description

External hemorrhoids are enlarged veins lying just under the skin, around the opening of the anus. There are also internal hemorrhoids inside the anal canal which lie under the rectal mucosa. Veins are fragile, thin-walled blood vessels returning blood back into the circulation after it has released oxygen and nutrients and collected cellular waste products. They are normally under low pressure compared to the thick-walled arteries, which are under higher pressure. Because of their thin walls they are susceptible to any increased pressure occurring when their drainage pattern is interfered with. In this particular area, they act like a balloon, increasing in size and shape and forming little bluish-colored sacs around the anus.

Hemorrhoids occur commonly in women, partially because of the effects of pregnancy. The enlarging uterus causes increased pressure within the pelvis, blocking some of the drainage from the rectal area, increasing the pressure within the vein. This increased pressure causes swelling and distention of the rectal veins, producing a hemorrhoid. In fact, this increased pressure is true for any region below the waist, including the pelvic and leg veins. This mechanism is discussed in more detail in the chapter on varicose veins (see p. 101). At the time of delivery, the pressure from the baby's head causes more obstruction to these veins. This, coupled with the increased abdominal pressure of bearing down, further distends the veins. With the birth of the baby the obstruction is removed and the pressure released, allowing the veins to shrink, but usually not to their original size. With subsequent pregnancies this process repeats itself, only now the tissues previously stretched have lost some of their elasticity. This puts them in a weakened state, allowing further stretching. Of course this doesn't happen in all cases, as there are many women who have borne children and show no signs of hemorrhoids.

Obviously there are other mechanisms for development as men, children, and women who have never been pregnant also develop hemorrhoids. Constipation with straining at stool for long periods or the pressure of lifting heavy objects are examples of other causes. Hemorrhoids are usually painless—the complications of hemorrhoids cause the discomfort: small sores (anal ulcers) or cracks in the lining of the anal canal (anal fissures), painful tunnels from inside the rectum draining out around the anus (fistulas) or blood clot formation in a hemorrhoid (thrombotic hemorrhoid) causing marked inflammation and pain.

Symptoms

One of the symptoms of hemorrhoids is the discovery of bright red blood on the toilet tissue after a bowel movement. On more rare occasions there can be active bleeding from the rectum to the point of making the patient anemic. Pain and itching in the rectal area are also common complaints. Some patients feel a mass in the rectal area which is actually hemorrhoidal tissue. An internal hemorrhoid can be pushed down by a piece of stool and prolapse (fall or slip out of place) out the anal canal. It is sometimes necessary for the patient to push this hemorrhoid back up into the anal canal to relieve symptoms.

Nonsurgical Treatment

If not too severe, hemorrhoids can be treated with stool softeners to relieve the straining during bowel movements.

Many of the mild symptoms can be relieved by sitting in a shallow pool of warm water (sitz bath). The hemorrhoids can be injected with a sclerosing agent which tends to reduce their size. Internal hemorrhoids can be removed by the doc-

> We should all give thanks to our skin each morning, for without it we would not only look funny but would soon be overrun by infection.

tor placing a rubber band tightly around the base of the hemorrhoid, thus shutting off the blood supply to the hemorrhoid and causing the tissues to die and slough off. The area will then usually heal without incident. Fissures sometimes respond to glycerin suppositories which melt, lubricating the rectal canal and allowing the stool to pass with less irritation.

Advertised ointments and creams which contain local anesthetic agents and anti-inflammatory agents numb and reduce swelling and inflammation. These measures are temporary and effective only if the condition is mild. Anesthetic drugs rubbed on the skin (topical) are only minimally effective, because the skin acts as the body's first line of defense. Skin has the ability to kill germs and act as a tough outer coating, preventing injury to underlying structures. We should all give thanks to our skin each morning, for without it we would not only look funny but would soon be overrun by infection. As germs and thorns find it difficult to penetrate the intact skin, so do the locally applied anesthetic drugs. A big problem, always, in self-medication is that a serious medical problem could be overlooked. In my years of practice I have seen more than one case in which a patient's self-treatment delayed diagnosis and effective treatment of a rectal cancer. The early symptoms can be very similar and impossible for the patient to differentiate.

The Laser

If there is currently a magic word in medicine it is *laser*. While most people are unaware of what a laser is, they feel it is the latest technology and want it used in their surgery. The word *laser* is an acronym for Light Amplification by Stimulated Emission of Radiation. A laser emits high-intensity light (or radiation) of one color in almost parallel waves. This concentrates much power in a small area. As a cutting tool, the laser has certain advantages over the scalpel. It can cut a finer line and seals the blood vessels as it cuts, limiting bleeding. The depth of the surgical cut can be accurately controlled, causing less trauma to the adjacent tissues and subsequently less pain and swelling. It is delicate enough to be used inside the eye and strong enough to remove hemorrhoids.

As with most good things, there are also disadvantages. The physician must have special training in the use of the laser to be granted laser privileges in most hospitals. The laser machine is expensive and the surgical personnel in the room must wear protective glasses. Despite these facts, many physicians are buying lasers for use in their offices.

In the surgery center where I practice we are doing hemorrhoidectomies on an outpatient basis. The patient is sedated and a long-acting (six-hour) local anesthetic is injected into the hemorrhoidal areas, which are then removed with a laser. The patient goes home, usually pain free, one hour after surgery. He will, of course, have pain when the local anesthetic wears off, but by then he will be home in his own environment and taking pain pills. So what once required a five-day stay in the hospital can now be done as an outpatient.

Surgical Procedure

There are many surgical techniques to remove hemorrhoids, but basically the aim is to disrupt the blood supply to the affected area and remove the redundant hemorrhoidal tissue. The nurse puts the patient's feet up in stirrups (the

> What once required a five-day stay in the hospital can now be done as an outpatient.

position used for female pelvic exams) with his bottom at the edge of the operating table. Other surgeons prefer the knee-chest position with the patient face down on hands and knees.

With the patient under anesthesia, the surgeon grasps the hemorrhoid with a clamp and cuts along its sides until it is freed from the rectal tissues. To make these incisions he may use a scalpel, cautery (electrical burning) or a laser. He now sutures the cut sides together, leaving a small opening for drainage. He repeats this for all the involved areas (usually there are three), always being sure to leave islands of normal tissue between excised areas so this normal tissue can spread and reduce scar formation. Fistulas are removed by passing a thin metal probe into the tunnel made by the fistula and excising the roof of the tunnel. This allows the fistula to heal from the bottom up. The patient can obtain prompt relief from a thrombotic hemorrhoid by having a surgeon open up the inflamed hemorrhoid with a small incision and squeeze out the clot. I can see you wincing. It's bad, but not that bad, because a little local anesthetic is injected into the affected area first. If left untreated the clot will eventually be absorbed and the symptoms will gradually disappear.

You may wonder how this area of the body can be operated on without the patient acquiring an infection from the

> The sigmoidoscope is a broom handle–sized, hollow, rigid tube about two feet long with a light on one end and a glass eyepiece on the other.

constant contamination of bowel movements. The answer lies in the fact that there is a very generous blood supply to the rectum which helps greatly in killing bacteria. By not closing the wound completely, leaving an area of drainage in the incisions, fluid will not accumulate and act as a home in which bacteria can grow and multiply.

As frightened as some patients are of having a hemorrhoidectomy, they are even more frightened of their first postoperative bowel movement. However, the doctor will give them stool softeners which cause a formed, soft and slippery stool. It is possible there will not be any greater discomfort (we are not allowed to use the word *pain*) during bowel movements than was experienced prior to surgery. The surgeon will also recommend soaking the area in a warm tub of water, which cleans the operative site, reduces discomfort and promotes healing.

Before starting the surgical procedure, your doctor will first do a digital exam of the lower rectal area by inserting his finger in the anus and feeling for any lesions. Then by inserting a sigmoidoscope through the anus into the rectum, he can see inside the lower large bowel. The sigmoidoscope is a broom handle–sized, hollow, rigid tube about two feet long with a light on one end and a glass eyepiece on the other. The eyepiece is removable so the surgeon can pass instruments through it with which to operate. As it is closed by the eyepiece on one end and inserted in the rectum on the other, it is airtight inside the tube, enabling the examiner to pump air through the sigmoidoscope and into the bowel. This air distends or opens up the walls of the colon for better visibility. The sigmoidoscope allows viewing and diagnosis of many unsuspected lesions of the colon. It is an important adjunctive diagnostic and therapeutic tool as small tumors can also be removed through it, thereby avoiding major surgery.

KNEE ARTHROSCOPY

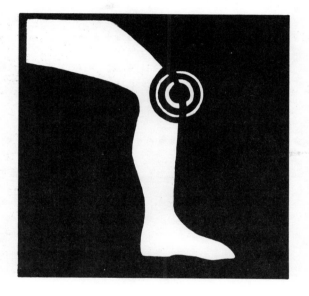

We see knee injuries in people from all walks of life, including the sedentary individual.

Description

The knee is a wonderfully designed joint for walking, running, sitting and getting us from one place to another. Unfortunately, the tremendous stresses we place on it during these everyday activities make the knee very susceptible to injury. To put it in perspective, every pound you weigh is magnified four to seven times within the knee during certain activities. A 200-pound man climbing stairs, for example, could exert pressures of over half a ton on the surfaces within the knee.

The upper leg bone, the femur, and the two bones of the lower leg, the tibia and fibula, are covered at the ends by a tough, resilient coating of cartilage. The pressures generated within the knee joint would damage this cartilage if it were not for the menisci. These small, flat, crescent-shaped cartilaginous disks lie between the upper and lower bones of the leg, one on each side of the knee, absorbing the shock and stress applied to the knee joint. With normal wear and tear these structures become worn and frayed, but continue to preserve the integrity of the joint.

Still, as simple an action as stepping off a curb and twisting your knee can generate enough pressure to tear a meniscus, and once torn it can become lodged in the joint, preventing complete extension of the knee. This is a painful condition and prevents normal walking. The torn edges can dig into the ends of the bones, causing pain and damaging their smooth surfaces, or cause enough irritation to the lining of the joint to produce excessive amounts of fluid. This excess fluid accumulates in the knee, causing swelling. If a misstep can cause this much of a problem, imagine what a forceful injury can do.

Prevention and Diagnosis

Although there is no absolute method of preventing injury to the knee joint, two factors may help reduce the risk: maintaining normal weight, and good muscle tone.

Because weight placed on the knee is magnified many times, the fewer extra pounds you carry, the less wear and tear there will be on the menisci and cartilages.

The bones of the knee joint are held tightly together by ligaments, which prevent the bones of the upper part of the leg from sliding around over the bones of the lower part of

> A 200-pound man climbing stairs could exert pressures of over half a ton on the surfaces within the knee.

the leg. By staying in good physical shape, with good muscular tone, you give support to the knee joint. This lessens the possibility of stretching these ligaments to the point where they can no longer properly support the knee joint.

In knee injury, a careful history and physical examination is the first order of business. If this does not provide adequate information, x-rays are taken. Magnetic resonance imaging (MRI) is also a valuable aid, as it shows tissues missed by conventional x-rays. (MRI aligns the electromagnetic charges of the area to be viewed in one direction and translates these electromagnetic charges into a very clear picture.) The meniscus is a good example of a structure not shown on x-ray, but well demonstrated by MRI. The ultimate diagnosis is made by looking into the knee joint with an arthroscope and viewing all surfaces.

Water on the Knee

In medical school there was the joke about the athlete who had water on the knee. He was negotiating a new five-year contract and didn't want the team owner to know about his disability. So he told his doctor to keep it a secret, because he didn't want it to *leak out*. However, it is not only the professional athlete who develops knee problems, nor the weekend jogger or tennis player. We see knee injuries in people from all walks of life, including the sedentary individual. Knee surgery is the most common type of surgery performed at the surgical center where I am medical director.

History

As little as ten years ago, knee injuries were treated by wrapping the knee with an elastic bandage or putting it in a brace. For an effusion (fluid within the joint), a needle was inserted into the joint and the fluid drawn off to relieve the pressure and soreness. Occasionally cortisone was injected into the joint to help keep fluid from accumulating again.

If a torn meniscus was suspected, open-knee surgery (arthrotomy) was performed. With the patient under anesthesia, the knee was surgically opened through a rather extensive incision. Using a knife specially designed to fit into the tight joint spaces, the involved meniscus was removed. This lengthy surgery was followed by three to five days in the hospital, during which the patient usually required injections of narcotics to control pain. The leg was placed in a large, bulky dressing which limited any motion of the knee joint for six weeks. Immobilizing the leg for this length of time causes joint stiffness, which worsens with age, and considerable atrophy (shrinking) of the leg muscles. It can take months of physical therapy to regain full range of motion in the knee joint, along with exercise to strengthen the leg muscles.

Obviously, this was a very debilitating surgery, requiring many months of hard physical therapy to regain full motion and strength in the leg. More important still, all of the involved meniscus was removed, not just the torn portion. Without the protective cushioning of the meniscus, wear and tear on knee joint surfaces is accelerated. This can lead to arthritis of the involved areas, with swelling and pain, and possible total knee joint replacement.

Surgical Procedure

The orthopedic surgeon still uses all of the above procedures; however, arthrotomy is far less common today. We now have a much more sophisticated method of viewing and operating on the knee.

For years urologists have been looking into the urinary bladder through long, hollow tubes called cystoscopes. A light on the end of the cystoscope allows illumination of the surgical field, and it has openings through which the surgeon inserts his instruments. Modifying, expanding and updating this technique has led to the development of the arthroscope.

In the arthroscope, the light bulb has been replaced by light-carrying fibers (fiber optics) which allow a very bright light outside the knee to be carried into the knee joint. A small television camera replaces the human eye at the viewing end of the arthroscope, and the surgeon performs the operation by watching the pictures the camera transmits to a TV screen. Many types of knives and other cutting instruments have been developed which can be inserted into the knee through incisions so small they usually don't have to be sutured closed. There are also motorized rotating blades

> A small television camera replaces the human eye at the viewing end of the arthroscope, and the surgeon performs the operation by watching the pictures the camera transmits to a TV screen.

(shavers) that act like miniature lawn mowers, trimming off any ragged edges of tissue.

After the patient is anesthetized, the surgeon makes three or four quarter-inch incisions around the knee. He passes an arthroscope through one of these incisions and surgical instruments through another. The third incision is connected by tubes to water bags, which are higher than the knee. The solution, forced by gravity into the knee, pushes the soft tissues away, opening up the inside of the knee for better viewing. By moving the arthroscope around, the surgeon can examine all portions of the knee joint. In fact, the contents of the knee can actually be viewed better by this method than when it is surgically opened.

If a torn meniscus is found, only the damaged portion is removed, leaving the remaining normal meniscus to protect the joint. Roughened areas within the knee are smoothed using the shaver. If a piece of cartilage or bone has been chipped loose, it is easily removed with a grasping forceps. Any area that has eroded through the cartilage to bare bone is filed down to encourage new blood supply and develop a fibrous coating. Once destroyed, cartilage will not regenerate, so a fibrous coating over the bone is better than exposed raw bone. At the end of surgery the knee joint is thoroughly flushed with fluid to remove any tissue fragments. The incisions are covered with small Band-Aids, and an elastic stocking is placed on the leg from toes to mid-thigh.

In our area this operation is performed as an outpatient procedure. The patient is admitted to our surgery center an hour before surgery and appropriate laboratory studies are performed. Next the patient is taken into surgery, where a general anesthetic is administered. After surgery—it takes approximately one hour—the patient is moved to the first-stage recovery room for an hour to recover from the anesthetic. Next comes a wheel chair ride to the second-stage recovery room. After sitting in a reclining chair for another hour, the patient walks out on crutches. Usually only moderate discomfort is experienced and oral medication may be taken for pain.

By comparison, arthroscopy makes arthrotomy appear to be something out of the dark ages. One is a fairly major surgery, with accompanying pain, hospitalization, disability and possible subsequent arthritis. The other is a short outpatient procedure, preserving as much normal tissue as possible.

As a bonus, orthopedic surgeons often connect a video recorder to the television camera at the end of the arthroscope and videotape the surgery. On the first postoperative visit the patient can see for himself the damage within the knee and the procedure that corrected it. "One picture is worth a thousand words."

APPENDECTOMY

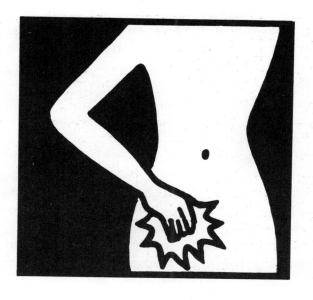

Because of its varied symptomatology, little progress has been made in the accurate diagnosis of appendicitis.

Description

The complete name of the appendix is the vermiform appendix. *Vermiform* means wormlike, and that is an accurate description of the way the appendix looks. It is a hollow muscular tube approximately three inches long and a quarter-inch wide. One end is attached to the colon where the small and large bowel join together. The opposite end is closed, forming a long, thin pouch. It is usually located in the right lower quadrant of the abdomen. A remnant of the development of the intestinal tract, the appendix has no known function. In fact, its removal does not seem to have any adverse effect on the body. This is why, given the potential development of appendicitis, it is not uncommon to remove a normal appendix during the course of an unrelated abdominal surgery. As long as the surgeon is in the vicinity, it is felt, why not take it out and eliminate possible future problems.

Appendicitis, an inflammation of the appendix usually caused by obstruction and infection, is treated by appendectomy, the surgical removal of the appendix. Though most common in adolescents and young adults, appendicitis can also occur in infants and the elderly.

The muscular walls of the appendix are capable of expelling the secretions produced from its lining, as well as plugs of digestive waste that collect within its cavity. If the appendix becomes unable to clear its cavity of an obstruction, the pressure created by the continual secretions will encourage bacterial growth and weaken its walls. This increased pressure can cause the walls to rupture (perforate), gradually allowing the infected contents of the appendix to leak into the abdominal cavity. Bacteria can become walled off and cause a local abscess or peritonitis—infection of the lining of the abdomen. Both conditions are serious and require surgical intervention. As wonderful as antibiotics are, they will not cure appendicitis without the source of infection being removed. Some people have survived perforation of the appendix without surgery because the infected area became walled off by intestinal tissue, but such cases are relatively rare.

Prevention and Diagnosis

Medical science has been able to do little to reduce the incidence of appendicitis; however, it has decreased in the

> Very bizarre and seemingly unrelated symptoms can sometimes be caused by appendicitis...partially because the tip of the appendix can be lying in any one of many different areas of the abdomen.

twenty-year period from 1940 to 1960, possibly due to the use of antibiotics. Because of its varied symptomatology, little progress has been made in the accurate diagnosis of appendicitis. The textbook case of right-lower-quadrant abdominal pain, increased white blood cell count, low-grade fever, nausea and vomiting makes the diagnosis seem quite a simple matter.

But doctors often see some or all of these symptoms in a person who has previously had his appendix removed—the moral being that the classic picture of appendicitis might represent any one of a number of different diseases.

On the other hand, very bizarre and seemingly unrelated symptoms can sometimes be caused by appendicitis. This is partially because the tip of the appendix can be lying in any one of many different areas of the abdomen, and the specific symptoms a patient experiences are in part related to the inflammation of the adjacent tissues which become involved.

For example, inflammation from an infected appendix might irritate the diaphragm—a large, flat muscle that separates the abdomen from the chest. Because of the distribution of nerves of the diaphragm, the pain is felt in the shoulder. This scenario (which I have personally seen) mimics a gallbladder attack—upper abdominal pain radiating to the right shoulder.

And I have also seen patients with minimal symptoms, who do not appear very ill, turn out to have far advanced disease. As you can see, diagnosing appendicitis can be very difficult and frustrating.

The Watermelon Seed Theory

Your mother may have told you that appendicitis was caused by swallowing watermelon seeds, which then became lodged in the appendix. According to this theory, there should only be appendicitis in watermelon season. Although there is now feeling in the medical community that appendicitis 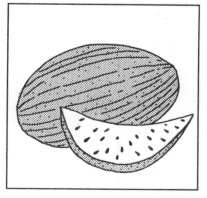 can indeed be caused by an obstructive mechanism, the watermelon seed theory has not yet been accepted.

Surgical Procedure

Removing the appendix is usually a simple matter of making an incision, called the McBurney skin incision, over the appendix. Next the surgeon dissects down, separating fat and muscle until he reaches the lining of the abdominal cavity. Great care must be taken not to lacerate the intestines when entering the abdominal cavity. If cut, the bowel contents could drain into the abdomen, causing infection.

Once inside, the surgeon locates a portion of bowel, frees it, and then gently removes it from inside the abdomen. Yes, that's right, a portion of the bowel is lifted out of the body and placed on the sterile drapes covering the patient. It is covered with moist towels to prevent the delicate tissues from drying out. This allows the surgeon to examine a large portion of the intestine to ensure that no other disease is

> Yes, that's right, a portion of the bowel is lifted out of the body and placed on the sterile drapes covering the patient.

present, as it is certainly possible to have more than one disease process going on at the same time. To find the appendix, he follows the small bowel down to where it joins the large bowel. He frees all adhesions until the appendix is attached only at its point of origin on the colon. The blood vessels feeding the appendix are tightly tied with sutures and then cut away from the appendix. Two thick sutures are tied near one another at the base of the appendix and it is removed by cutting between the sutures. One suture is left on the colon, closing the hole made by the removal of the appendix. This keeps the colon from leaking its contents into the abdominal cavity. Finally, the intestinal contents lying on the drapes are carefully placed back into the abdomen before closing.

Wrong 20–30 Percent of the Time

If after surgery your surgeon should tell you your appendix was normal and he could find no cause for your symptoms, don't jump to the conclusion that he slept through "Stomach Aches" in medical school. Rather understand that, given certain symptomatology, your doctor *must* suspect appendicitis.

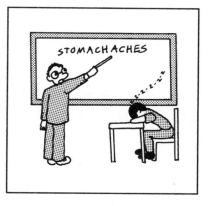

There are no absolute tests for appendicitis; its diagnosis is based on the summation of many factors. Surgical exploration is the only way to know for sure. Your doctor must play Sherlock Holmes, trying to deduce which are pertinent findings and which are the red herrings that tend to confuse the investigator. After all, the physician is in many ways a detective, sifting through facts and trying to properly interpret them. He uses the medical laboratory much the way Holmes used Scotland Yard's criminal lab. The body can be just as devious an opponent to finding the cause of an illness as the most elusive criminal. And the stakes are equally high, for a perforated appendix is a life-and-death situation.

STERILIZATION

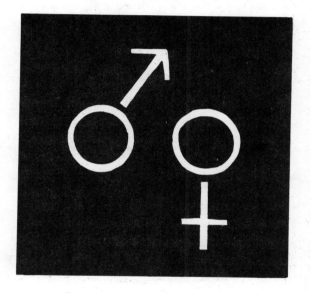

It is potentially a far more serious condition to enter the abdominal cavity for tubal ligation in the female than to enter the scrotal sac for vasectomy in the male.

Description

The process of fertilization of the ovum by a sperm is a complex procedure and an interruption in any part of this mechanism will be effective in preventing pregnancy from occurring. To understand how the different methods of contraception work, I think a little review of the reproductive process is in order. The ovaries produce an ovum (egg) once a month which ruptures free from the ovary. It is picked up by the "fimbriated" end of the fallopian tube which has tiny fingerlike projections that sweep the egg into the fallopian tube. The sperm is produced in the testicles of the male where it passes through tubes and out the end of the penis during intercourse. The sperm is deposited in the vagina where it travels up through the uterus into the fallopian tube where fertilization takes place. The fertilized ovum now moves down into the uterus where it attaches to the side of the uterine wall. Here it makes its home and here is where it stays during pregnancy.

Nonsurgical Treatment

The most natural method of birth control is the rhythm method: having intercourse during that part of the menstrual cycle when pregnancy can't take place. Many people use this method; however, you may have heard the question: What do you call people who use the rhythm method of birth control? The answer: Parents. While this system of birth control has worked for some, it has failed many others. Other nonsurgical methods of birth control—the pill, condom, intra-uterine device (IUD), vaginal foam and diaphragm—are well known to most people. But there are reasons why some people don't want to use these forms of birth control. For some it is the potential complications of the birth control pill, or infection and unwanted permanent sterilization caused by certain IUDs, or the high failure rate that forces them to look for another method. For others it is the loss of spontaneity of having to prepare a contraceptive device prior to intercourse. There is much material on these subjects in the lay journals; here we will discuss the surgical procedures available for both men and women.

Surgical Procedure for Men: Vasectomy

This is the only surgical sterilization technique available today for men. Vasectomy is a simple, inexpensive and safe operation entailing the tying off of the tubes carrying sperm from the testicles to the penis. It is done in the surgeon's office with the patient going home after surgery. Postoperatively there is minimal discomfort and moderate swelling of the testicles.

To perform a vasectomy the surgeon, by palpation, locates the proper tube (ductus deferens) and injects a local anesthetic agent into this area. This is usually the only part of the surgery that causes any discomfort. A clamp is placed on the skin and around this tube to keep it from slipping away and having to be relocated. He dissects through skin and connective tissue until he comes to the tube and surgically removes a short section. He ties a suture around the end of this tube which connects into the penis so no sperm can accidentally enter—or exit! The other end, which comes from the testicle and contains sperm, is sewn into a different layer of tissue. This end of the tube is not sutured shut so sperm being produced can still travel out of the testicle.

With this method there is no back pressure or any abnormal change in the testicle. The continuity of the tube has been interrupted and the two ends are in different tissue plains, with the end going to the penis sutured shut. This technique does not stop the production of sperm; it merely interrupts its flow to the penis. The sperm produced are deposited in the soft tissues of the scrotum and absorbed by the body. As there are two testicles, this procedure is repeated on the opposite side. For the male to be considered sterile he must undergo several sperm counts postoperatively until it is shown positively that no sperm are left in the ducts. Also, there can be auxiliary ducts not seen during surgery which can carry the sperm to the penis. It is important to use some

> Vasectomy does not affect the sensation of sex or ejaculation, but the semen contains no sperm.

form of birth control until a satisfactory sperm count is obtained.

Vasectomy does not affect the sensation of sex or ejaculation, but the semen contains no sperm. One major drawback of surgical sterilization is that it is considered permanent. Some can be reversed, but some cannot. While it takes thirty minutes to perform a vasectomy, it requires about four hours to try and effectively sew the cut ends back together for vasectomy reversal. While reversal is not always successful, many are; my own grandson is the result of one example.

Surgical Procedure for Women: Tubal Ligation

This is the female equivalent of the vasectomy. The fallopian tubes connect the inside of the abdomen with the outside world. The 200 million to 300 million sperm deposited in the vagina during intercourse try to wiggle their way up through the cervix into the uterus. From here they enter the fallopian tubes which connect to the upper part of the uterus. The ovum enters from the other end of the fallopian tube and makes it way toward the uterus. Out of the millions of sperm deposited in the vagina only a few hundred get close to the egg, and only one fertilizes it. After the egg is fertilized by one sperm the door is shut and no more sperm can penetrate the outer coating of the egg. The egg and sperm meet and join forces within the fallopian tube and move on into the uterus where they hope to find a home.

By interrupting the opening through the fallopian tube anywhere along its path, this meeting can be prevented. No meeting, no pregnancy. Since the fallopian tube is entirely within the abdominal cavity, this cavity must be entered to reach and tie off the tubes. Yes there are two tubes, one on the right side of the pelvis and one on the left. The ovaries have the same layout and both tubes must be ligated, as monthly ovulation takes place alternately between the two sides.

Many women elect to have their tubes tied just after giving birth. At this time the uterus is still very large. The fallopian tubes which normally lie at a level below the pubic hairline are now even with the belly button. Under anesthesia it is a relatively simple matter to make a small incision around the belly button and dissect down into the abdominal cavity. Once inside the abdomen the fallopian tubes can usually easily be found coming off the upper sides of the uterus. One at a time they are grasped with a forceps, a suture is tied around them in two spots, and the in-between section is removed. Now when the ovum is present during intercourse, it will be on one side of the missing section and the sperm will be on the other. This procedure adds very little, if any, to the postpartum recovery time.

Most tubal ligations are performed at a time other than delivery. There are several approaches to entering the abdominal cavity, and the approach dictates the name of the procedure.

Vaginal Tubal Ligation

In vaginal tubal ligation the incision is made through the blind end of the vagina. Using a speculum to hold the vagina open, the surgeon makes a small hole in the end of the vagina and looks into the abdominal cavity. Using long instruments he can find and grasp a fallopian tube, tie it off and remove a section. He then repeats this on the other side. The vaginal incision is closed and the whole procedure, assuming all goes well, takes only thirty minutes. Sometimes, due to adhesions or other causes, one or both tubes cannot be found and the surgeon can't complete the sterilizing procedure by this technique.

Laparoscopic Tubal Ligation

With the development and popularity of medical scopes, we also have the laparoscopic tubal. Here a long, thin needle is inserted into the abdominal cavity near the belly button and carbon dioxide gas is pumped into it. This causes the abdomen to become distended and swell to the size of a six-

or seven-month pregnancy. Now a small incision is made at the belly button and a pencil-sized trocar (a hollow, sharp needle) is inserted rather blindly into the abdomen. The purpose of the gas is to keep any bowel or other important structures out of the way of the needle. A laparoscope, which is similar to an arthroscope (see Knee Arthroscopy, p. 32), is inserted through the trocar. By direct viewing the tubes are found and, using special instruments, clamped, clipped, cut or cauterized.

The sterilization technique is the same as other approaches, with the tubes being cut in two and the ends clipped or cauterized closed. The gas is allowed to escape through the trocar, and the abdomen again regains its normal shape. The laparoscope is removed and the small incision repaired. Because the pressure exerted by the gas pushes the diaphragm up and compresses the lungs, it requires a more complicated type of anesthetic (see Anesthesia and Monitoring, p. 6).

Abdominal Tubal Ligation

The older, traditional method, which is still in use today, is to make a small abdominal incision just above the pubic hairline and dissect down into the abdominal cavity and perform the ligation through this incision.

All tubal ligations involve entering the abdominal cavity. In most cases these surgeries are performed without any major complications. However it is potentially a far more serious condition to enter the abdominal cavity for tubal ligation in the female than to enter the scrotal sac for vasectomy in the male. Even so, tubal ligation continues to be a popular surgery.

OPEN-HEART SURGERY

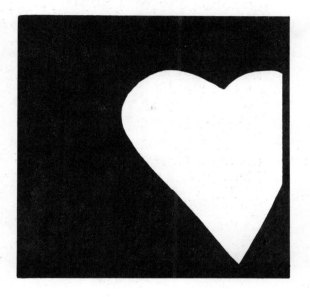

It is absurd to wait until you have a heart attack, as so many people do, before changing to a more healthy diet and life style.

Description

The status symbol of the sixties was the Cadillac car, in the seventies it was the Mercedes Benz. But in the eighties, it's the unbuttoned shirt showing an open-heart surgery scar running down the middle of the chest. There have been great advances made in the field of heart surgery in the last few years. Today a wide array of medical and surgical treatments are available to the heart patient. When I started in medicine almost thirty years ago we had little in the way of surgery to offer the patient with heart disease.

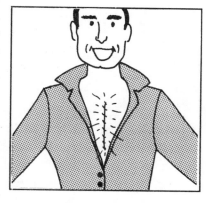

The heart is made up of four chambers surrounded by the heart muscles, which must be nourished with oxygen. As the average heart beats seventy times each minute, these muscles must contract more than once every second. I'll leave the math to you as to how often your heart beats in a year. Needless to say, there is a large and constant demand for oxygen requiring a continuous flow of blood to these muscles. This is accomplished by small blood vessels (coronary arteries) which carry blood to all parts of the heart muscle.

In hardening of the arteries (arteriosclerosis) the passageways through the coronary arteries become narrowed with plaques and less blood is able to pass through to the heart muscle. If the supply of oxygen decreases below a certain point, but is still adequate to sustain the life of the heart muscle, you get aching of the heart muscles (angina). This is a warning that the blood supply to the heart is not adequate

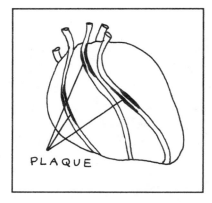

PLAQUE

to meet its metabolic needs. If the blood supply is further decreased to the point that an area of heart muscle can't survive, it dies. This is a heart attack (myocardial infarction)—often a sudden and fatal event.

Death is frequently caused by a sudden shock to the heart that makes the heart muscle beat in a nonorganized manner. This random contracting (ventricular fibrillation) of the heart muscles is not effective in propelling the blood out of the heart. It is more of a twitching of the heart muscles than a contraction and has no force to push the blood into the circulation. Many people, if given effective cardiopulmonary resuscitation (CPR), will again develop an effective heart beat and survive their heart attack. This is because the damage to the heart is not incompatible with life, but the onset of ventricular fibrillation is. If CPR is given until a counter electric shock (defibrillation) can be administered to restart cardiac contractions, the heart attack victim has a good chance to survive.

Diagnosis

The electrocardiogram (EKG) is very helpful in determining if there is any damage to the heart, but it gives us very little information as to the specific condition of the coronary arteries. The definitive test of their condition is the coronary artery angiogram. A hollow wire is inserted into an artery and threaded up into the heart. Once in proper location a radiopaque dye (it shows up on x-rays) is injected through the wire. This dye goes into the coronary arteries and x-ray pictures produced on a fluoroscopy screen show the degree of blockage and its exact location in the coronary artery. A motion picture camera records these x-ray pictures so there is a permanent record of the findings. This allows doctors to carefully review them and even to freeze the pictures at a critical time for more detailed examination. With the patient and his family also viewing the films, they have a better understanding of the problem.

Nonsurgical Treatment

As the cause of coronary artery disease is the slow process of hardening of the arteries, the preventive treatment starts years before the problem begins. Newspapers, TV and magazines are full of stories relating heart disease to high cholesterol levels, obesity and smoking. It is absurd to wait until you have a heart attack, as so many people do, before changing to a more healthy diet and life style. The medical literature is filled with articles relating smoking to many medical problems, including heart disease, yet 30 percent of the adults in this country smoke. The first line of preventive treatment is a healthy diet, no smoking, and exercise. Of course there are other factors: heredity and genes. But since we had no choice in the selection of our parents and grandparents, there is nothing we can do but play the hand we have been dealt.

There has been an explosion of new cardiac medications to control the symptoms of heart disease. Many have the ability to reduce the oxygen requirements of the heart muscles, while others have the ability to increase the blood supply to the heart. One of the new and exciting medical treatments for a heart attack is to inject a thrombolytic agent into an arm vein which dissolves the obstruction in the coronary artery. If this is done before it has a chance to destroy any of the heart muscle, the heart can survive without damage. In fact, the new generation of cardiac drugs are so improved there are many doctors who feel medical treatment can be as effective as surgical intervention.

Angioplasty

The coronary arteries usually get blocked in small segments, so it was only a matter of time until a nonsurgical method was devised to unblock these segments. Now it is possible to insert wires through the groin or arm into an artery and thread it backward into the heart. Under direct x-ray vision the wires can actually be directed into the obstructed coronary arteries. The wire is inserted into the partially blocked area and a small balloon on the end of the wire is inflated. As it inflates, the balloon stretches the constricted area of the coronary artery, breaking down the plaques and relieving the blockage. The amount of pressure within the balloon can be carefully controlled so there is less danger of over-inflating it and damaging the artery.

This procedure is called an angioplasty and is performed in the hospital by a cardiologist with the patient under local anesthesia. As inflation of the balloon may further decrease an already compromised blood supply, it is important that the patient be awake to relate any symptoms. If the procedure is successful, the patient frequently can go home the following day. With the advent of angioplasty, the number of open-heart surgeries being done has greatly decreased. It is a far simpler procedure than open-heart surgery, with fewer risks and hardly any discomfort; but, unfortunately, it is not appropriate for all patients.

Lasers have found their way into many specialty fields of medicine, including cardiac surgery. Although not yet widely used, they show great promise in their ability to clear the plaques out of obstructed arteries, and in time lasers could replace the inflatable balloon now used in angioplasty.

History

The first corrective operation for heart disease in which I participated was called the Vineberg Procedure. In this operation one end of an artery was taken from the chest wall and sewn into the heart muscle. It was thought this would bring new arteries into the heart muscle. This operation was performed for many years until studies showed improvement was no greater than when surgically opening and closing the chest without operating on the heart. Any improvement was apparently just a placebo effect—due to psychological causes, not medical. This is not an isolated occurrence; many medical conditions have been found to improve with a sugar pill.

The Heart-Lung Machine

Open-heart surgery requires the surgeon to sew arteries and tissues that lie directly on the heart. This would be very difficult if the heart were beating. A mechanism was needed to allow stoppage of the heart and still have profusion of blood to all organs. This became possible with the development of the heart-lung machine, which takes over the pumping action of the heart and the ventilation of the lungs.

The heart, for all practical purposes, is divided into a right and left side. The right side takes blood that has been depleted of oxygen and nutrients and pumps it to the lungs where it is oxygenated and cleared of waste products. The left side of the heart takes this oxygenated blood and pumps it to all parts of the body. It requires much greater pumping action to distribute blood to the body than to the lungs, resulting in the left side of the heart being larger and more

> Since the left side of the heart has more muscle mass, it also requires a greater blood supply. It is no wonder, then, that it is also the side that has the most problems.

powerful. Since the left side of the heart has more muscle mass, it also requires a greater blood supply. It is no wonder, then, that it is also the side that has the most problems.

The heart-lung machine is connected to the patient's circulation by plastic tubes inserted into the right and left sides of the heart. The one to the right side of the heart carries blood away from the patient into the heart-lung machine, while the one connected to the left side carries blood to the body from the heart-lung machine. Besides circulating the blood, the heart-lung machine passes oxygen through it before returning it to the patient. The blood is also cooled to lower the body's temperature and reduce its requirement for oxygen. Once connected to the heart-lung machine, the heart beat and breathing can be stopped, as the heart-lung machine is performing these functions.

The heart will continue to beat, however, if not artificially stopped. This can be accomplished in several ways, but usually it is by an infusion of a cold solution of drugs into the heart. This now gives the surgeon the ability to do his very delicate surgery on a still heart, with the additional benefit of the heart muscle resting and requiring less oxygen. One of the wonderful things blood knows to do is to clot when it leaves the confines of the vascular system. Therefore an anticoagulant drug is given to prevent clotting of the blood inside the plastic tubes of the heart-lung machine. This is good in that it prevents the blood from clotting outside of the body, but bad in that it also prevents clotting in the surgical site. Naturally this increases bleeding in a procedure which already involves substantial blood loss. To help control this problem, some of the suctions used to clear the blood from the surgical area are connected to another machine called a cell saver. As you can guess from its name, it collects and cleans the blood cells, which can then safely be given back to the patient. This is far safer than giving banked blood, as this is the patient's own blood and there is no danger of hepatitis, AIDS or incompatible blood reactions.

Surgical Procedure

Coronary artery bypass graft surgery (CABG) has proven to be a useful tool in improving the quality of life and increasing longevity in patients with coronary artery disease. In some medical centers it has evolved into a routine and relatively safe procedure. Reasons for this improvement are the development of newer surgical techniques, better drugs, more sophisticated monitoring, more experienced surgeons and in-depth understanding of the dynamics of the heart.

The skin incision is made down the center of the chest to the breastbone (sternum), which is split with an electric saw. As the heart and major blood vessels lie directly below this area, care must be taken not to accidently damage them. A large metal retractor is inserted between the cut sides of the sternum, forcing the edges apart. Bleeding is stopped and the lining around the heart (pericardial sac) is opened, exposing the heart. The involved coronary arteries are located and

> The skin incision is made down the center of the chest to the breastbone (sternum), which is split with an electric saw.

exposed for grafting. A generous incision is made in the calf of one leg to facilitate removal of a long strip of vein. This vein will have several branches which must be sutured closed. If these communicating veins are not properly sealed off, the vein will leak when used as a graft. One end of a portion of this vein is sewn onto the main artery coming out of the heart (aorta), and the other end into the coronary artery past the obstructed area. Now when the heart beats, the blood goes from the aorta through the vein graft, bypassing the obstruction into the opened section of the coronary artery. From the coronary artery it can now flow unobstructed to the heart muscle.

This process is repeated for all of the involved coronary arteries (there can be as many as six), each time using another piece of the leg vein. If the surgeon runs out of vein, he will harvest one from the other calf. As difficult as this surgery is, one of the more challenging problems is to make the vein grafts the proper length. If the graft is too long it could kink and obstruct, and if too short it could tear loose from the heart. One reason this is not as simple as it would seem is that the vein is capable of changing its length after being cut by going into spasm. If the coronary arteries are blocked their entire length, there is no portion of the coronary artery to graft to that is open enough to allow blood to flow into the heart muscle. In these cases CABG is of no value.

Grafts can remain open indefinitely or they can close up after a very short period of time. They tend to develop the same disease process that affects the coronary arteries. In these instances, the patient may require another CABG or possibly an angioplasty to reestablish adequate blood supply to the heart.

GALLBLADDER SURGERY

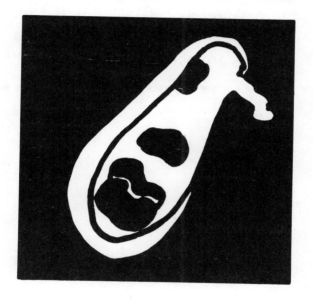

Approximately 500,000 gallbladder surgeries costing a total of a billion dollars are performed each year.

Remember how your favorite movie cowboy would walk into the local saloon, place his foot on the bar railing and order a whiskey? He would then drop his prospector's pouch of gold nuggets on the bar to pay for a round of drinks. Remember that pouch—it is the size and shape of a gallbladder. Your cowboy had something good in his pouch, but the person with gallbladder disease (cholecystitis) has only worthless gallstones (cholelithiasis). Well, not completely worthless, as they represent quite a few dollars to the medical community. Approximately 500,000 gallbladder surgeries costing a total of a billion dollars are performed each year.

Description

The gallbladder lies under the lower edge of the liver, which is roughly even with the lower part of the rib cage on the right side. This is convenient because the bile, formed in the liver, has only a short distance to travel to reach the gallbladder. Gallbladder pain is usually felt in the right upper quadrant of the abdomen. I say usually, because the body has a remarkable ability to refer pain to other areas. The sensation of pain is carried from nerve endings via nerve fibers to the brain, which then interprets where the pain originated from. Most nerves pass through several areas of the body, sending off branches to these areas. When these branches are stimulated by pain sensation, the brain can become confused as to the origin of this painful stimulation. It can interpret the pain as coming from an adjacent uninvolved area.

An example would be the phantom limb pain (pseudesthesia) of an amputated arm. Pain is perceived as coming from the missing hand because the nerve that supplied the hand is receiving pain stimulation on its course from the point of amputation to the brain. The brain knows this nerve went to the hand and interprets the pain as coming from there. Likewise an inflamed gallbladder can cause irritation to the diaphragm which can refer the pain to the right shoulder. So the presenting symptom could be right shoulder pain even though the inflammation is in the abdomen. Most of the time the brain is not fooled and you hurt where the problem is. I think these examples will help the reader appreciate the difficulties this trick of nature gives your physician in trying to make a diagnosis.

Fair-Fat-Forty-Female

In my day, all medical students were taught the four F's of gallbladder disease. Therefore when a Fair, Fat, Forty-ish Female came into my office (I was in general practice for six years) complaining of headaches, sore throat, ear aches or leg pains, I always thought of gallbladder disease. I've never forgotten the puzzled expressions on their faces when I would suggest gallbladder x-rays. I subsequently learned that you must have a few more symptoms of gallbladder disease to make the four F's significant.

Diagnosis

Diagnosis of gallbladder disease starts with the same steps as most other diseases: a good history and physical examination. A history of right-upper-quadrant abdominal pain, nausea, fever, and fatty-food intolerance would be strongly suggestive. On physical examination the area over the gallbladder is tender to palpation, but the gallbladder can be felt in less than half of the cases. X-rays of the gallbladder after ingestion of oral dye (oral cholecystogram) will usually

demonstrate gallbladder disease if present. This was once
the common definitive test
for gallbladder disease, but it
has largely been replaced by
ultrasonography. Ultrasonography uses ultrasound
waves and has the advantage
of requiring no x-rays or
dyes. It is excellent in demon-
strating gallstones or gallbladder disease.

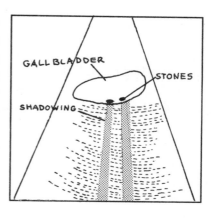

What's It For?

Obviously your gallbladder isn't a pouch for holding
gold nuggets, but what is it for? Is it some apparently worthless organ Mother Nature put in the body like the appendix?
No, it collects the bile formed in the liver, changing it from a
thin, watery liquid to a thicker, more concentrated and bio-
logically active form. The bile is stored in this concentrated
form until you bite down on fried chicken or other fatty
foods. This causes the muscles within the walls of the gallbladder to contract, forcing the bile out through a narrow
duct which empties into the small bowel. Here the bile attacks the fats and breaks them down to smaller, more easily
absorbable particles.

If you have a gallbladder full of stones this duct can
become plugged, and when the gallbladder squeezes down
in response to a fatty meal, it can't empty because of the
blockage. The pressure within the gallbladder increases and
you get colicky pain in the right upper quadrant of the abdomen. This obstruction can be complete, with the bile stagnat-

ing and the walls of the gallbladder becoming inflamed. You now not only have pain, but fever, nausea, vomiting and generalized debilitation.

Another complication of a completely plugged bile duct is that the bile being formed has no place to go. It is then absorbed into the blood stream, imparting a yellowish color

> Gallstones can be large or small, few or many, and range from gravel size to that of an avocado seed.

to the skin and organs of the body. This is one of the causes of yellow jaundice. It will disappear when the obstruction is removed and the bile can again drain into the intestinal tract. The patient will then get his rosy pink color back, provided he had a rosy pink color before he got jaundiced. You can tell if a non-Caucasian is jaundiced by examining the whites of his eyes. If they are yellow, he is jaundiced, as this area of the eye around the pupil is normally white in all races. Gallstones can be large or small, few or many, and range from gravel size to that of an avocado seed. They develop from the cholesterol and other chemicals present in the bile.

Nonsurgical Treatment

The simplest treatment which is sometimes helpful is to change diets and avoid fatty foods. In some cases it is possible to avoid surgery by doing this, but there is risk of a gallbladder attack at any time. There are some people who discover they have gallstones while being tested for other diseases. It is not uncommon for them to show up on x-rays of the abdomen taken for reasons completely unrelated to the gallbladder. They have no symptoms from their gallstones and could continue symptom-free for the rest of their lives. The decision to remove the gallbladder on a person without any symptoms is a difficult one and is best made on an individual basis.

As is common in medicine, a technique developed for one application can find use in another unrelated field. The machine used to fragment kidney stones and allow them to harmlessly pass out through the urine has been used to re-

> Once you have recovered from surgery, there are no dietary restrictions.

move gallstones. A machine called a lithotriptor sends out ultrasound shock waves and breaks the gallstones into small pieces which can then pass out through the bile ducts. At first glance this technique seems to have a tremendous advantage over surgery. It is essentially a nonsurgical procedure, with far less pain and recovery time. It is not widely used, however, because the gallbladder is diseased, and removing the stones and leaving the gallbladder won't keep them from recurring. Additionally, some small fragments of stones could still cause an obstruction in the gallbladder ducts.

There are also drugs that can be taken by mouth which will dissolve some gallstones. The problem here again is that the stones tend to re-form, and the medication must be taken for long periods of time. The internists and surgeons I know overwhelmingly recommend surgical removal of the gall-bladder for stones or inflammation.

Surgical Procedure

The surgeon makes an incision in the right upper quadrant of the abdomen just below the rib cage. He carefully dissects through fat and muscle layers down to the liver. Peeking out from under its edge is the blind, or closed, end of the gallbladder—remember, it's like a pouch. The open end connecting to the liver is buried down under its edge. He

> The internists and surgeons I know overwhelmingly recommend surgical removal of the gallbladder for stones or inflammation.

grasps the blind end with a clamp, and dissects the gallbladder off the underside of the liver. When he gets to the narrower base of the gallbladder he ties off the ducts and cuts them in two so he can remove the gallbladder.

Now you say, "Dummy, how am I going to eat fatty foods? I couldn't eat them before, because they gave my gallbladder fits. Now there's nothing to squish down and hurt, but there's also no bile to aid in digesting the fat." Well, the main duct from the liver to the intestinal tract was intentionally left intact by your surgeon. This duct will enlarge until it is able to take over the functions of the gallbladder, allowing you to once again enjoy your gastro-epicurean delights. In fact, once you have recovered from surgery, there are no dietary restrictions.

Getting back to the surgery, the surgeon checks all of the bile ducts to ensure that no stones have become lodged in them. If stones are present they must be removed. One way to tell if stones are present at the time of surgery is by injecting a radiopaque dye (it shows up on x-rays) directly into the ducts while they are exposed. Once all stones have been removed, he sews up the raw undersurface of the liver where the gallbladder was attached. This prevents adhesions from forming or bleeding from developing. He now sutures the corresponding layers of tissues together, and then closes the skin. A sterile dressing is placed over the wound and the patient is taken to the recovery room.

CATARACT SURGERY

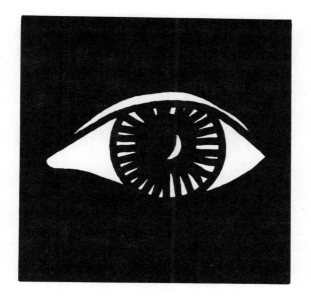

Cataracts can be congenital (you are born with them), but the degenerative form is more common. They also can be caused by diseases like diabetes or chronic use of medications such as cortisone.

Description

Textbook descriptions of the anatomy and function of the human eye always compare it to a camera, and with good reason. There are many similarities between the various parts of the eye and those of a camera. Any image must first pass through the pupil to enter the eye; in the camera this is the function of the shutter. As light falling on the eye increases, the pupillary size decreases to diminish the amount of light entering the eye. Dim light has the opposite effect—the pupil dilates to allow more light to enter. The camera shutter also has

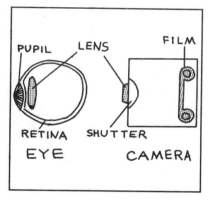

the function of adjusting the amount of light entering the camera and eventually striking the film. Too much light will overexpose the film and too little will underexpose it. The same holds true for the eye, with too little light causing a dim image. (Most people have had the experience of a doctor shining a light into their eyes during a physical examination. The bright light causes the pupil to constrict as it tries to limit the amount of light entering the eye. Doctors use this principle to check for certain types of brain injury which can interrupt this reflex.)

After entering the pupil (or shutter) the image next passes through the lens of the eye (or camera). Then it is projected in inverse fashion onto the retina of the eye (or the film in the camera). The retina, the lining of the back of the eye, is where the visual image is picked up by nerve cells and relayed to the brain. These electrical impulses are converted by the brain into the images we see. Even though these images are upside down on the retina, the brain turns them right side up without our realizing it. People need to wear glasses when the visual image is not sharply focused on the retina; the corrective action of glasses refocuses the image clearly. Just as you must focus a camera to obtain a clear picture, the lens of the eye must also constantly be focused. There are small muscles on each side of the human lens that adjust its shape to obtain a clear image. As you look from near to distant objects, the shape of the lens changes to obtain the best possible focus.

In the formation of a cataract the lens gradually becomes cloudy and then eventually totally opaque. As sight depends on the visual image passing through the lens onto the retina, this image is either distorted, blurred or else completely blocked. A simple comparison is to look through a very dirty window and see how distorted objects appear. This is a gradual, completely painless process, the only symptom being loss of visual acuity. This can happen so gradually that it often goes unnoticed by the patient until it becomes severe. A strange thing can happen during this process if the opacity is in a particular central portion of the lens. It changes the refraction of the lens enough to enable a farsighted person to become temporarily nearsighted and to read without glasses. This is called "second sight," but it wanes with the advancement of the cataract formation.

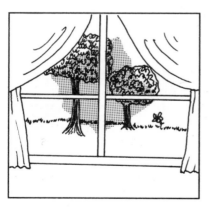

Cataracts can be congenital (you are born with them), but the degenerative form is more common. They also can be caused by diseases like diabetes or chronic use of medications such as cortisone. Most older patients' cataracts are caused by degeneration of the lens. The cause of this gradual cloudiness of the lens is unknown and there is no way to prevent its occurrence or to slow down its progression. Except for trauma to the eye, which can cause formation of a cataract, most other causes result in cataracts forming in both eyes.

When I started in medicine, cataract surgery required the patient to spend many days in the hospital with the head held very still between sand bags. Today cataract surgery is done on an outpatient basis with the patient going home shortly after surgery. Except for lifting, bending and straining, the patient is allowed to perform most activities.

Nonsurgical Treatment

The only nonsurgical treatment for cataracts is frequent refraction (examination) of the eyes with corresponding changes in the correction of the patient's glasses. This will sometimes help correct the visual disturbances in the early stages of cataract formation, but will not affect the progression or severity of the cataract.

Surgical Procedure

The purpose of cataract surgery is to remove the cloudy lens from inside the eye. As this is a painful procedure which involves making an incision in the eye and manipulating instruments within the eye, some sort of anesthesia is required. Luckily, this is easily accomplished by the injection of a local anesthetic agent behind the eye. A long needle is inserted next to the eye and advanced at an angle until it lies behind the eye. A small amount of local anesthetic is then injected, numbing the eye and causing temporary blindness. Because administration of the local anesthetic is painful, a small amount of intravenous anesthetic is administered just

> When I started in medicine, cataract surgery required the patient to spend many days in the hospital with the head held very still between sand bags.

prior to this injection. This renders the patient insensible for several minutes while the anesthetic block is being given. The patient awakens in a few minutes and the surgery can continue without any discomfort. As most cataract patients are in the older age group, this technique is easier and safer for them.

There are several methods of removing a cataract. The older technique involves making an incision at the junction of the white part of the eye (the sclera) and the colored part of the eye (the iris). Through this incision instruments are used to free the lens from its supporting muscles. Once freed from all connecting tissues, the lens is removed in one piece. This is accomplished by inserting a long, thin instrument with either a suction cup on its end which can be attached to the lens, or else a freezing probe that freezes itself to the lens. Both of these methods allow the lens to be pulled out of the eye easily.

The newer method of removing the lens is called phagoemulsification. In this method only a small incision is made in the eye and an ultrasonic probe is then inserted. This probe vibrates rapidly and breaks the lens into very small pieces which are then suctioned out of the eye. The advantage of this technique is that a small incision heals with less potential for problems. Both of these methods require the surgeon to perform delicate surgery on small structures within the eye, but with the advent of the surgical microscope it has largely become routine. The microscope magnifies all the intraocular structures, making it much easier for the surgeon to perform the surgery.

Until recently the post-cataract patient had to wear very thick glasses to compensate for the loss of the lens inside the eye. When not wearing glasses vision was limited—even getting up at night to use the bathroom entailed finding and putting on glasses in order to see. This was a significant limitation, particularly for older patients. With the advent of the intraocular lens (IOL) this became unnecessary. At the time of cataract surgery the IOL—a small, plastic artificial lens—is inserted into the eye behind the pupil. The lens is left in place for the life of the patient where it usually causes no problem. This immediately partially corrects for the loss of the real lens and gives the patient functional vision; however, glasses or contact lenses are usually required to obtain maximum visual acuity. Patients who have had cataracts removed prior to the advent of the IOL can have one inserted as a secondary surgical procedure.

LOW BACK SURGERY

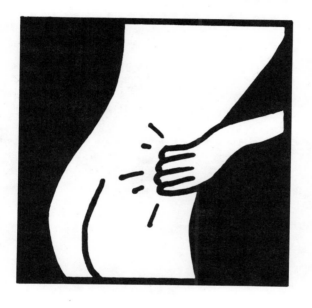

Back problems are extremely
common, with over 5 million
Americans disabled each year
at a cost of over a billion dollars.

Description

The spine, which starts below the head and continues to the bottom of the lower back, is made up of vertebrae. These bones, round in the front with projections on each side in the back, contain the circular canal through which the spinal cord passes. Foramina (holes) in the side of each vertebral body allow nerves to pass through. Intervertebral disks lie between the vertebrae and act as shock absorbers. They are round and flat with a tough outer coating and gelatinous center. If the outer coating of an intervertebral disk becomes weak or ruptures, the inner material can herniate (bulge out), pressing on nerves. It is this pressure on the nerves passing out of the vertebral foramina that causes symptoms. Usually it is the lumbar (low back) vertebrae which are affected.

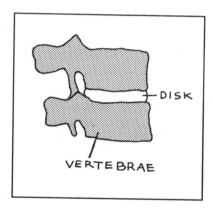

Back problems are extremely common, with over 5 million Americans disabled each year at a cost of over a billion dollars. Some authorities estimate that more than 80 percent of the population will experience significant back pain sometime in their adult life.

The onset of low back pain can be sudden and severe—set off by nothing more than bending over to pull a weed out of a flower bed—or it can have a gradual and insidious onset. Most people have low back pain for many years before they develop pain radiating down into their legs. As with so many disease states, the symptoms of herniated lumbar disk can vary greatly. Where symptoms are experienced depends on the level of the herniation in the low back, because the nerves exiting from each level of the spinal cord go to different parts of the body.

I have jokingly asked new nursing students why a giraffe has such a long neck. They usually answer, "Because he has many more vertebrae in his neck than we do." The truth is, giraffes and humans have the exact same number: seven. (I tell them the reason for the giraffe's long neck is that his head is so far away from his body.) I mention this to illustrate that things are not always as they appear. The leg pain or numbness experienced by patients with a herniated disk does not originate in the leg, but rather in the low back. There is nothing wrong with the nerves or muscles in the leg.

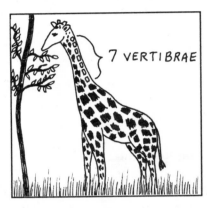

7 VERTIBRAE

When the pressure on a nerve is great enough to interrupt its function, permanent damage to that nerve can result. If the damaged nerve is one that controls the contraction of a muscle (a motor nerve), then that muscle will not respond properly to impulses sent to it from the brain. One relatively common example of this is what is called a foot drop. The nerve controlling the muscles that lift the front of the foot off the ground in walking is damaged, and to take a step the foot must be lifted by the leg high enough in the air to clear the ground. See for youself how this works: Take a few steps with your foot pointed down. You will quickly realize that you raise your foot to a horizontal position with each step.

Diagnosis

Diagnosis of herniated lumbar disk is made from a combination of patient history, physical examination and x-rays. The symptoms can vary from minor discomfort in the low

> Newer x-ray procedures have the remarkable ability to manipulate images three-dimensionally using computers.

back to excruciating pain. This pain can be so severe that some patients feel they are paralyzed and can't move. The expression "paralyzed with fear" should be, in this case, "paralyzed with the fear of *pain*"—the pain that will be caused by any movement of the legs or back. Many patients give a history of some manner of bending activity that they associate with the onset of their pain. This pain can be confined to the back or it can radiate down the front or back of the leg, and it can also be associated with numbness or weakness. Frequently, when the pain starts radiating down the leg the back pain disappears. The pain is exaggerated by any maneuver that increases the pressure within the spinal canal, such as sneezing, coughing or any type of straining. A test as simple as having the patient lie flat on his back and raise one leg in the air, which stretches the nerve and exacerbates the pain, can further confirm the diagnosis. Usually there is ample time after diagnosis to attempt conservative (nonsurgical) treatment, but one of the more serious and urgent symptoms—urinary retention or incontinence (loss of bladder control)—demands immediate treatment.

In the past the only x-ray that would definitely confirm a ruptured disk was a myelogram, for which a dye that shows up on x-rays is injected into the spinal fluid. This could cause a severe headache after the procedure, or a reaction to the dye could cause later problems, such as increased back pain. Conventional x-rays of the back do not show the spinal canal or the vertebral disks. With the advent of the CAT scan and magnetic resonance imaging, however, the myelogram is no longer necessary to make a diagnosis. These newer x-ray procedures have the remarkable ability to manipulate images three-dimensionally using computers. For example, x-rays of the spine taken from the side can be made to appear as if taken from above looking down on the vertebrae. They also show the soft-tissue structures not seen on conventional x-rays.

Nonsurgical Treatment

There is much controversy regarding surgical and conservative treatment of herniated lumbar disk. It was thought by some experts that the only adequate treatment for herniated lumbar disk was surgical removal of the disk. Today, however, the more prevalent theory is that conservative therapy offers equally good or better results in some cases.

Conservative management encompasses a combination of many different modalities of treatment. There is a wide divergence among doctors as to what types of treatment offer the best chance of improvement for the patient.

The first and probably the oldest treatment is bed rest. Some doctors treat the patient initially with complete bed rest, except for bathroom privileges, for a week or two. This can be done in the patient's own home if the family is cooperative and understanding. Other doctors feel that bed rest is counterproductive, causing weakness and loss of minerals from the bones, and complete bed rest is not recommended. In fact, one orthopedic specialist I heard lecture allows jogging very shortly after the onset of acute symptoms.

> Other doctors feel that bed rest is counterproductive, causing weakness and loss of minerals from the bones.

Almost all of the doctors prescribing conservative therapy recommend some sort of physical therapy. This may take the form of lying in bed with traction or mild exercises to build up the strength of the back muscles. The mainstay of conservative therapy is the administration of an assortment of pharmaceutical agents. The anti-inflammatory drugs come in steroidal and nonsteroidal forms. The first are the cortisone-like drugs; the latter range from the very mild, such as aspirin, to more potent types. Both the steroidal and nonsteroidal anti-inflammatory drugs can have different but significant side effects.

Along with one of the anti-inflammatory drugs, muscle-relaxing medications are also commonly prescribed. Their effectiveness may be related to their sedating and tranquilizing effects rather than their actual ability to relax the spasmodic muscles. Patients also usually need some sort of pain-relieving medication. Because the pain can continue for a protracted period of time, most doctors use nonnarcotic pain relievers to help avoid any form of drug addiction.

If these measures fail to provide relief, the patient can be hospitalized, where treatment can be more closely controlled. At this point it is not uncommon to have an anesthesiologist administer a series of cortisone-like injections through the back into the area of the herniated disk.

Twenty years ago a new and simple method, injecting the vertebral disk with a substance called chymopapain, was first tried. The chymopapain had the ability to dissolve the nucleus of the herniated disk, relieving the pressure on the nerves and alleviating symptoms. As this is a very simple procedure when compared to back surgery, it held great promise as an alternative to surgery in certain selected cases. In fact, the beneficial results proved to be very favorable when compared to back surgery. Unfortunately, some very serious and even fatal allergic reactions to chymopapain have caused most surgeons to stop using it.

If significant symptoms persist after conservative treatment, then surgical intervention can be considered. The patient must have a thorough understanding of what his condition is likely to be with continued conservative therapy and what he can reasonably expect his results to be with surgery. He should further understand that, except for some specific conditions, this is an elective surgery and does not have to be performed.

Surgical Procedure

Almost any type of anesthesia can be used, including local, spinal, epidural and general. This choice varies widely from one area of the country to another. After administration of anesthesia the patient is turned face down on the operating room table. Great care must be taken to ensure that no parts of the body are placed in unnatural positions that could produce injury while the patient is anesthetized. The low back is then prepped with an antiseptic solution and sterile drapes are arranged around the surgical site. An incision is made over the affected area and continued down to a tough fibrous layer (ligament) that surrounds the vertebrae. To identify the exact level of the spinal cord that he is operating on, the surgeon may insert a needle into the area and check

> The patient should further understand that, except for some specific conditions, this is an elective surgery and does not have to be performed.

its location by x-ray or use certain structures as landmarks. He opens up the ligament with a scalpel to expose the vertebra beneath it. Then with a bone-biting instrument he removes part of the vertebra, making access to the intervertebral disk and the nerve coming out of the vertebra. Irritation of this nerve by a herniated disk will be the cause of pain radiating down the leg. A long biting instrument is used to remove any tissue impinging on the nerve. It is important that this be done to ensure that there will be no further irritation to the nerve. Next the intervertebral disk is entered through an incision made by a scalpel and the inside is carefully removed using another long biting instrument. After removal of as much as possible of the intervertebral disk, the surgeon meticulously stops all bleeding. A small layer of fat is dissected off an adjacent area and placed over the operative site. Each layer of tissue is then sutured closed, including the skin. A sterile dressing is applied over the incision and the patient is taken to the recovery room, where he remains for approximately an hour before being transferred to his hospital room. The patient is encouraged to walk the day after surgery and usually leaves the hospital in five to seven days.

It is important for the patient to realize that although he may not have pain after surgery, his back will never be completely normal. He should be taught exercises to strengthen his back muscles and advised on the proper method of lifting.

LIPOSUCTION

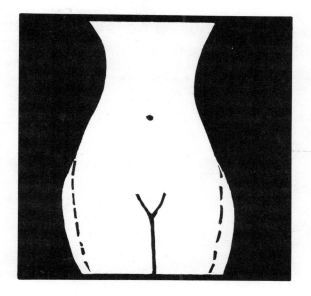

This is not a weight reduction
technique, but rather body
sculpturing.

History confirms that people have always been concerned about appearances. The ornate robes and jewelry found in archaeological sites and graves gives evidence to this fact. In some cultures people have physically altered their appearance, for example, the Ubangi women of central Africa whose lips are pierced and stretched around flat wooden disks. In this country the slim-and-trim look is what most people strive for, even though there is a natural tendency for fatpads to develop, especially below the waist. These unwanted fatpads are often inherited traits and can be seen on members of several generations of the same family.

For decades surgeons have been trying to surgically remove these and other unwanted fatpads from the body. There have been some successes, but also many failures. It is only within the last three or four years that a safe, effective and esthetically acceptable method has been available. For the patient with generalized obesity, there is still no simple surgical treatment. For these patients, there are major abdominal surgeries that affect the absorption of nutrients from the gastrointestinal track—serious surgeries, fraught with very significant medical complications. The less radical treatment of wiring the jaw shut so only liquids can be taken is simpler and safer, but it has met with only limited success.

Surgeons have had the technical skills necessary to remove unwanted fat from certain areas of the body for many years. The procedure entailed making very long incisions and surgically removing large sections of fatty tissue and skin. This resulted in large, unsightly scars which in part offset the benefit obtained by the fat removal. To avoid these scars some surgeons tried making small incisions through which they could scoop out the fatty tissue, but because this technique had many complications, it was not widely accepted. The main problem with this technique, though not recognized at the time, was its use of a sharp surgical instrument rather than a dull one. The sharper the instrument, the more it disrupted the blood supply, causing unacceptable amounts of bleeding.

Description

Liposuction is the removal of fatty tissue from the body by the use of a blunt cannula (hollow tube) connected to strong suction. This is not a weight reduction technique, but rather body sculpturing. Liposuction is not for the obese patient who wants to lose weight from all over the body. It is used, rather, for removal of fat from selected parts of the body. The most common area for liposuction in women is the so-called saddle bags on each side of the hips, while in men it is the "love handles" around the sides of the waist. Other common areas are the thighs, buttocks, abdomen, breasts, face and neck. The liposuctioning of breasts is not just for

> The body usually does not generate additional fat cells— that's the good news.

women—men with gynecomastia (large breasts) can benefit from it also. Liposuction is often performed in combination with other procedures, such as cosmetic or plastic surgeries, particularly around the eyes during a face lift.

Liposuction has proven to be an effective and safe procedure, so it is no wonder that it has grown rapidly in popularity. Besides obvious large fat deposits, there are smaller areas such as under the chin or around the ankles where excess fat can be removed with liposuction. The ideal patient for liposuction is a young, healthy person who has one or two areas of the body in need of reduction. This is a personal perception and, aside from the possible psychological implications, is of no medical significance. This is why insurance companies consider liposuction to be a cosmetic procedure and ordinarily exclude it from payment. Of course, this means that the patient must bear the entire cost of the procedure.

Goods News/Bad News

The basic premise of liposuction stems from the fact that we are born with a specific number of fat cells which, in most individuals, cease to multiply after puberty. These cells have the ability to increase in size, but not in number. By surgically removing them, the area involved has a reduced number of fat cells. The body usually does not generate additional fat cells—that's the good news. The bad news is that the remaining cells can enlarge in size if there is a weight gain. Some individuals do have the ability to produce additional cells, but they are usually grossly obese, and not candidates for liposuction. After the fat has been removed there is the problem of excess skin. In young people the skin is elastic and has the ability to shrink and tighten. In older people this elasticity is lost and the skin, without the fat beneath it, can become loose and flabby; thus liposuction was initially recommended only for people forty years old or younger. Today, with improved techniques, it is appropriate for all ages, as many older people are not concerned about loose skin that doesn't show; they are content to just have clothing fit and look good on them.

Nonsurgical Treatment

There is no nonsurgical way to remove fat from a particular place in the body. Machines that massage the behind, for example, will not remove fat from that area. Diet and exercise reduce the body's stores of fat, but not necessarily in the appropriate places. If there is weight loss, fat is often partially lost from the needed areas, but usually not a satisfactory amount.

Surgical Procedure

It is important that the patient have reasonable expectations of what liposuction can achieve. For example, cellulite probably won't be affected much by liposuction, as it is the deeper fatty tissue that is removed, not the more superficial layer that causes dimpling of the skin. So if a patient assumes that his cellulite will disappear, he will be unhappy with the results. Diet and exercise should be tried first to reduce certain areas of the body, not surgery.

It is also imperative that the surgeon carefully examine the areas to be treated before surgery, because he can't see the tissues he is removing during surgery and he must be certain that the protrusions are actual fatpads, not bony prominences or even bowel from an abdominal hernia. One of the basic principles of surgery is: if you can't see it, don't cut it. This led to a natural reluctance on the part of surgeons to accept a procedure that is done without any direct view of the tissues being removed.

Whether this procedure is performed using local anesthesia with sedation or using general anesthesia is determined by the areas to be liposuctioned and the amount of fat to be removed. After adequate anesthesia is administered and the surgical site is prepped and draped, a small incision is made. The site for these incisions need only be in the general vicinity of the fatpad, as the long cannula can reach into the nearby area. They can be made in natural creases or areas covered by underclothing and when healed they will be very inconspicuous.

Cellulite probably won't be affected much by liposuction, as it is the deeper fatty tissue that is removed, not the more superficial layer that causes dimpling of the skin.

A dull cannula is inserted through the incision into the area to be liposuctioned. A blunt cannula is used because it will push nerves and blood vessels out of the way rather than severing them. This minimizes bleeding during surgery and lessens the amount of postoperative numbness. It also dislodges the fat cells, allowing them to be more easily suctioned. A strong suction is applied to the end of the cannula and with long in-and-out motions the surgeon suctions the fat out of the affected area. Each in-and-out sweep of the cannula leaves a hollow track.

The cannula is held in one hand and the other is used as a guide to feel the skin and fat of the area being liposuctioned. This gives the surgeon some control over how much tissue is being removed, particularly important when one side must match an opposite side. If there is bleeding in any track the surgeon moves to another track, thereby decreasing the bleeding. There are limits to the amount of fat that can be

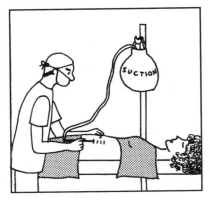

suctioned out at any one time. Up to 1500 cc (approximately a quart and a half) of material can be removed safely as an outpatient. Removal of larger amounts is probably best performed in a hospital. Besides blood loss, there is a large unseen loss of fluids called third spacing. This is the fluid that leaves the blood and cells to collect in the tissues between the cells. The loss of blood and fluid is compensated for by replacement with large volumes of intravenous solutions.

Postoperative bleeding and swelling are of vital concern, and because this is essentially a blind surgical procedure with no way to directly stop the bleeding, a tight dressing is applied to hold the tissues together, compress the blood vessels to stop bleeding, and prevent the formation of fluid under the skin. This excess fluid can cause a fibrous capsule to form, preventing the skin from attaching to the underlying tissues and resulting in unsightly wrinkles. Drains are inserted into larger areas so that any fluid will leak out around the drain and not accumulate in the tissues where it might cause infection. Antibiotics are also given to help prevent postoperative infections.

Because of swelling, the results of liposuction are not always apparent until several months after surgery. In fact, swelling can sometimes make the treated areas actually appear larger than before surgery, a very distressing situation for patients who have not been informed about it.

How often we have all heard someone say, "I wish I could take it off here and put it there," while pointing from their hips to their breasts. Well, there are doctors removing the fat from the hips or other areas by liposuction and injecting it into the breasts. This is not for breast enlargement, as breast implants are, but rather to add a little to one breast that might be smaller than the other. While it is conceded that about 50 percent of the fat cells will die, this still leaves 50 percent that will live. Smaller areas such as indented scars can also be injected with fat to raise them up to the level of surrounding tissues, and there is the added benefit of the donor site having been liposuctioned!

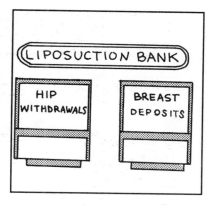

Liposuction is a new and controversial technique capable not only of reshaping the body but also of generating some serious side effects. Anyone contemplating this procedure would be well advised to obtain several opinions.

VARICOSE VEIN STRIPPING

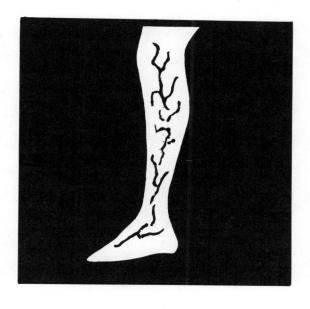

Varicose veins can be an unsightly condition but their appearance is not the primary indication for surgical removal in most cases.

Description

Twenty million people in this country are affected by varicose veins to some extent.

To understand the surgery for varicose veins, a little lesson in the anatomy of arteries and veins is in order. A vein is a thin-walled, rather fragile duct or tube which carries blood from outlying parts of the body back to the heart. Some veins are superficial and easily seen through the skin of most people; they are the bluish raised lines on the back of the hand or at the bend of the arm. In contrast, an artery is a strong, elastic, thick-walled vessel lying deeper under the skin and carrying blood away from the heart. While not visible, they can be located by feeling for their pulsations. A common example is your own pulse at the wrist, but there are many other places in the body where they can be felt. Oxygen and nutrients are carried to all parts of the body by the arteries, while the veins perform the opposite function— carrying the waste products of metabolism away from the individual cells. In this process oxygen is replenished and carbon dioxide is removed.

The term *varicose veins* is used to describe that condition of the legs where veins appear under the skin as large, bluish, wormlike lumps. Although common in men and in women without children, it is most prevalent in the female who has borne children. The enlarged uterus fills the pelvis and compresses the blood vessels in this area. The veins do not have the pressure of the pumping action of the heart pushing the blood through them, as the arteries do, making the veins very susceptible to compression and blockage by increased pelvic pressure.

There are small check valves within the veins of the legs. Their purpose is to reduce the effective length of the column of blood in the leg by breaking it down into shorter seg-

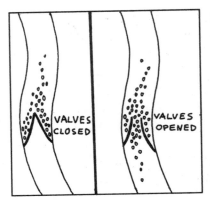

ments. With the valves, you only have the pressure of each section between the valves exerting pressure on the vein walls. When these valves become stretched or incompetent, the column of blood becomes longer, increasing the pressure within the vein and causing it to stretch.

Remember that veins are thin-walled and fragile. Increased pressure within the vein forces the fragile vein wall to stretch, increasing in both width and length. As the leg is only so long and these veins can't hang down below the foot, they become tortuous; that is, they twist and turn to accommodate the increased length. Another important effect of the increased pressure is that it causes the veins to dilate. The veins are now not only longer, but are also much wider with a larger cross-sectional diameter. Instead of a few straight, smooth, firm and invisible veins running up the leg, there are now many large, sacular, lumpy, dilated veins traveling in all directions across the leg. An example of the dilating effect of obstruction to veinous blood flow is when your doctor puts a tourniquet around your arm before taking a blood sample. The tourniquet blocks the flow of blood out of the vein, but since blood is still coming into the vein this increased pressure causes the vein to enlarge, making it easier to puncture with a needle.

Varicose veins can be an unsightly condition when the legs are exposed by dresses, shorts or a bathing suit. But their appearance is not the primary indication for surgical removal in most cases. Varicose veins are unable to properly carry waste products back to the heart because their long and tortuous route recirculates the blood in the leg rather than directing it back toward the heart. Some of the waste products diffuse out into the tissues of the legs causing itching and discoloration. This discoloration can progress to the point of breaking down the tissues of the skin, causing an ulcer to form. These ulcers become infected easily and, because of the

> Varicose veins are unable to properly carry waste products back to the heart because their route recirculates the blood in the leg rather than directing it back toward the heart.

stagnation of circulation in this area, heal poorly. With the accumulation of waste products in the leg muscles, they begin to ache, cramp and feel tired.

These are serious complications, but they pale in comparison to the most feared complication of all—pulmonary embolism. The tortuosity of the veins slows the flow of blood, which can cause it to sludge up and clot. This blood clot normally will remain in the leg, but it can become dislodged and travel up the course of the vein toward the heart. From here it can go to many places, but wherever it lodges it will obstruct the blood flow to that area. If it goes through the heart into the lungs, it can and frequently does cause sudden death. This is called a pulmonary embolism and was much more common when patients were kept in bed for prolonged periods after childbirth or surgery.

The flow of blood through the veins back to the heart depends in part on the squeezing of the veins by the movement of the leg muscles. Inactivity and subsequent slowing of the blood flow in the legs, even without varicose veins, can cause clots. This is one reason patients are now encouraged to walk as early as possible after surgery. It is such a serious concern that some surgeons actually give drugs prior to surgery that inhibit clotting of the blood; it has been found that small doses of these anticoagulant drugs decrease the incidence of postoperative blood clots without increasing the surgical blood loss significantly.

Nonsurgical Treatment

The simplest and least expensive treatment is to get off your feet several times a day and elevate your legs above your heart. This lets gravity reduce the pressure inside the vein, causing it to empty more completely. Another simple treatment is wearing elastic stockings or bandages on the leg. The pressure of the stockings, being greater than the pressure within the vein, forces the blood out of the vein. Without any blood in the vein it collapses, halting any further degeneration. This blood is redirected through communicating branches into the veins deep inside the middle of the leg. These deep veins do not become tortuous as they are supported by the muscles of the leg.

This in no way cures the varicose veins, but it relieves symptoms and reduces the possibility of complications. If the varicose veins are not too advanced, a sclerosing agent can be injected directly into them. This material is so irritating that it causes inflammation and blood can no longer flow through them. One of the complications of this form of treatment is that if the sclerosing solution should leak out of the vein, it could adversely affect the surrounding tissues.

Surgical Procedure

In surgical removal, the surgeon does an amazing thing. He violates the surgical principle that an incision heals from side to side, and not from end to end. According to this principle a very long incision will heal just as fast as a short one, because it is the cut edges that come together to heal and not the opposite ends. Since some of the leg veins run from the ankle to the groin, it would take a very long incision to surgically remove them. Of course the larger the scar the larger the surgical fee, so it is much to the surgeon's credit that he doesn't make one incision down the entire length of the leg. What he does instead is substitute an ingenious technique which, on paper, sounds barbaric but works very well.

A small incision is made at the ankle and another in the groin, both over opposite ends of the greater saphenous vein. Cutting into the vein at the ankle, the surgeon inserts one end of a thick, flexible wire (strip-per) into the cut end of the vein. After insertion, the stripper is threaded all the way up the vein to the groin. He ties the cut end of the vein at the ankle securely to the stripper. The stripper now lies under the skin and within the walls of the greater saphenous vein from the ankle to the groin. Grasping the end

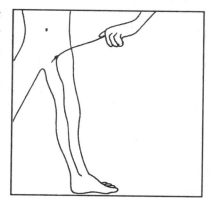

of the stripper at the groin, with a firm steady pressure, the surgeon pulls on the stripper until he has pulled it all the way out of the leg. This doesn't sound so bad, until you remember that he tied the other end of the stripper to the vein at the ankle. So when the stripper is pulled out of the leg, the end of the vein at the ankle necessarily must follow. Since this is one long continuous vein it is pulled out of the leg from the ankle to the groin. This vein is like a tree with many connecting branches which are at first stretched and

> This vein is like a tree with many connecting branches which are at first stretched and then ripped off from the main vein as it is progressively removed.

then ripped off from the main vein as it is progressively removed. The process of tearing continues for the entire length of the leg and terminates only after all branches have been torn off.

This technique works well for long, relatively straight veins; however, most of the varicose veins of the leg are too tortuous to allow passage of a stripper through them. These are removed by making a small skin incision over each sacular, lumpy vein and dissecting down to where it can be grasped with a clamp. By blunt dissection the vein is freed a short distance along its course, then it is also ripped out. By removing segments of the vein the flow of blood is interupted, and without a source of blood, the vein will no longer be able to fill. It will then collapse and lie flat under the skin. Finding and removing all the varicose veins can be a tedious and slow task. Even a moderately involved leg may need ten to fifteen of these incisions. When all the veins have been removed the skin incisions are individually sutured closed.

All the while, the doctor has given no thought to the bleeding that might be occurring from those torn, ragged ends of the veins left behind. That is, not until now, when it is Band-Aid time. He knows the family will judge his surgery by the size of the bandage, so he wraps the entire leg in an elastic bandage to make it look sick, which by now it is. It's hard to believe, but the snug elastic bandage keeps the bleeding and swelling controlled and consequently the pain also. The patient can ambulate (walk) the next day and usually requires only light pain medication. The skin incisions heal nicely and after several months the bermuda shorts can go back on.

With the veins gone, how is the blood going to get back up the leg to the heart? The veins removed were just under the skin and there are so many of these superficial veins (you can't see most of them) that it is of no consequence if a few are removed. These smaller remaining veins will enlarge to handle the flow of blood. In fact, they can and often do enlarge enough to become varicose veins themselves. This is why the condition can recur and require additional surgery.

HERNIA REPAIR

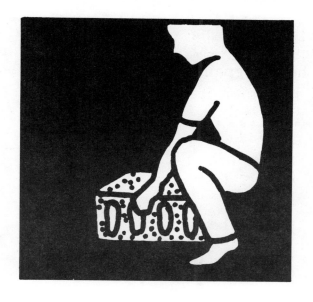

There are good reasons to have a
hernia repaired besides the physical
discomfort it might be causing you.

Description

A hernia is the abnormal protrusion of all or part of an organ through the containing wall of its cavity. Many places in the human body can develop a hernia. You can have something as simple as a muscle herniating out of its sheath to complex herniation of the stomach into the chest. This chapter deals with the hernia which occurs in the groin area, the inguinal hernia.

Hernias are more common in men than in women because of (1) the fetal origin of the testicles and (2) greater physical exertion. The testicles, which I hope everybody knows belong in the scrotum, start life in the abdomen. As the fetus develops, some unknown power pulls them down a tract into the scrotum, where they remain. The testicle, on its journey down the inguinal canal, must pass through some openings or rings. Occasionally, these rings do not close up tightly behind them, leaving a residual weakness which could allow the bowel to follow the testicle into the scrotum at a later date. The weakness can be severe enough to cause a hernia to be present at birth (congenital hernia), or it may take another fifty to sixty years of activity for a hernia to develop.

Just standing creates a great deal of pressure within the abdomen, which is increased by lifting, coughing or straining. Feel your abdomen the next time you are lifting, and you will get some idea of how tight the abdominal muscles can become. The abdominal cavity is closed on all sides so pressure applied to one side, such as lifting produces, increases the pressure within the cavity. It is this intra-abdominal pressure that pushes the bowel through the weakened area creating the bulge in the groin or herniation into the scrotum. Enough bowel can pass into the scrotum to greatly enlarge it, making walking difficult and uncomfortable. A similar weakness occurs in the female, caused by a structure called the round ligament, although there is, of course, no scrotum for the bowel to herniate into.

Sometimes the testicle doesn't want to leave the safe, warm confines of the abdomen, and stops on its way down to the scrotum. This is called an undescended testicle and leaves the scrotum void of that testicle. If not surgically repaired, there is a greater incidence of cancer or atrophy (shrinkage) of the testicle and loss of its ability to produce sperm.

Diagnosis

Usually the patient notes a swelling in the groin area when standing or straining that disappears when lying down. There may be pain associated with the swelling, or there may be pain and no swelling. The symptoms will frequently disappear on lying down because this reduces the intra-abdominal pressure, allowing the intestines to return to the abdominal cavity. Most men have had the experience of having a doctor put a finger up under their scrotum while being asked to turn their head to the side and cough. Coughing increases the intra-abdominal pressure enough to force the bowel down into a relaxed ring, were it can be felt by the doctor's finger. If the ring is tight and firm, this can also be felt. (You are asked to turn your head to the side, not because it helps in the diagnosis, but to keep you from coughing directly on the doctor—he doesn't want to catch your hernia.)

Inguinal hernias can be classified into three types, the simplest of which is (1) the reducible hernia, meaning the abdominal contents can be pushed back into the abdomen. This can become (2) an irreducible hernia by the formation of adhesions which may prevent its contents returning to the abdominal cavity. The most serious is (3) the strangulated hernia. This is when the blood supply going through the hernia is shut off, damaging the intestines. The treatment of inguinal hernia is surgical repair.

Nonsurgical Treatment

Grandpa knew how to treat his hernia. He would put on a truss—a belt worn around the waist with a knob attached to it which fitted over the hernial bulge. Pressure from the knob, being greater than the intra-abdominal pressure, would keep the hernia pushed in or reduced. There are good reasons to have a hernia repaired besides the physical discomfort it might be causing you. They never heal; the tissues become weaker and the hernia larger. With the intestines bulging out in places they don't belong, it is easy to get a kink in the intestinal tract, similar to the twisting of a garden hose. If you kink the bowel, the intestinal contents can't move down the intestinal tract and you have the very serious problem of a bowel obstruction, just as a kinked garden hose causes a water obstruction. If not corrected, this can become even more serious: You get swelling to the point that the pressure of the swollen tissues is great enough to squeeze the walls of the blood vessels together, shutting off the supply of blood to that segment of bowel dependent on them. With the blood supply decreased below the viable level, that segment of the intestines will die; and if something isn't done promptly, so will you.

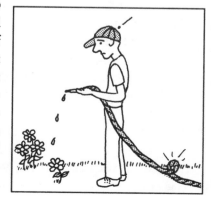

Surgical Procedure

The groin area is prepped by shaving off any hair and scrubbing with an antiseptic solution. The reason that hair is always shaved from a skin incision area is that hair can't effectively be washed clean. Sterile drapes are placed all around the operative site. Following the prep and draping, a skin incision is made in the groin area where the hernia originates. The surgeon carefully dissects through skin, fat and muscle, avoiding important structures—particularly, in

> The reason that hair is always shaved from a skin incision area is that hair can't effectively be washed clean.

the male, the spermatic cord (a tube that transports sperm). At the hernia site there is a hernial sac. This sac is made of peritoneum (the lining of the abdominal cavity) and may contain intestines or other abdominal contents. Common ones are omentum, which is a fold of peritoneum containing fat or, in young girls, an ovary. The surgeon locates the hernial sac, frees it up and places any of its contents back into the abdominal cavity. If intestines are present they are carefully examined to make sure they are viable (able to live). Also, all tissue replaced is checked for active bleeding, which might have been caused when freeing them from adhesions. He then ties off the base of the hernial sac and cuts off the remainder.

The inguinal ring is then sutured snug, bringing good, strong supporting tissue over the weakened area. Since the blood supply to the testicle goes through this ring, it must not be sewn so tight as to interfere with it. Loss of the testicular blood supply would destroy the function of that testicle. The kicker is that if it isn't sutured tightly enough the hernia will recur. If the tissues are too thin or fragile, the surgeon may sew in a nylonlike mesh to strengthen the repair. He then closes each layer with suture until he is back to skin, which is also sutured closed.

The Kinked Garden Hose Syndrome

Now, if the patient was foresighted enough to have this surgery when it was a simple hernia, that would be all there is to it. It takes about one hour to perform the operation. But if he decided to let it go, and developed the kinked garden hose syndrome, he could have real problems. If the bowel is damaged beyond the point where it can recover after unkinking, it must be resected out. This is a bowel resection, which requires the surgical excision of the damaged portion of bowel and is a much more serious operation than just doing a hernia repair. It is as if you cut a section out of your garden hose and now have to sew the cut ends together. This must be done in such a manner that the ends won't leak, or cause an obstruction due to formation of scar tissue. And after the bowel resection is done, the hernia must still be repaired.

By the time the patient gets to the hospital and into surgery, he is not in the same physical condition as the person who hasn't procrastinated. With a bowel obstruction the patient can become dehydrated from vomiting and fever, and toxic from bowel contents leaking into the abdominal cavity. When performed electively, hernia repair is a less serious operation done on a healthier patient. All that is gained by waiting is that the patient will stay out of the hospital a little longer, but stay in a lot longer. "Well," you say, "I'm not going to do either one. When Grandpa passed away, he left his truss up in the attic and I'm going to wear it." Go ahead, but the constant pressure of the truss against an already weakened area will only further weaken these tissues. The truss doesn't cause anything to heal and must be worn the rest of your life. Who wants to spend the rest of his life with a belt around his hip and a door knob poking him in the gut? Because that's pretty much what a truss is, a belt with a big knob on it. Are you also going to go to bed with the truss on? Because you can strain in bed, too, unless you're older than Grandpa was when he died.

Inguinal hernias can be repaired under local, regional or general anesthesia. The type I like best is local anesthesia with sedation. The patient is given short-acting sedation, while the surgeon injects a long-acting local anesthetic solution into the operative site. The patient is asleep for this potentially painful experience, so he feels no discomfort. He is then allowed to gradually awaken while the operation is under way. If at any point during the surgery the patient should feel pain, more of the local anesthetic is injected. When the operation is over, the patient can walk to the recovery room and be discharged from the facility an hour later without any discomfort.

An undescended testicle can be surgically corrected by loosening up its attachments and pulling it into the scrotal sac. It must be sutured in place or it tends to return to its former position. Sometimes the testicle can't be brought down into the scrotum for anatomical reasons or because it has been previously surgically removed. This gives the scrotum an empty, deflated appearance, making some men self-conscious. A scrotal implant can be surgically inserted into the empty scrotum, restoring normal appearance.

HYSTERECTOMY

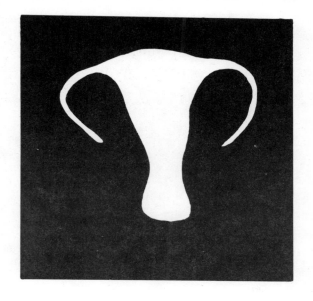

One-third of all women in
this country will have a
hysterectomy by age 65.

Description

Of all the marvelous wonders of nature, the reproduction of human life is to my mind the most amazing. The uterus is a prime player in the game of feeding and housing a newly conceived life. It must prepare for the possible implantation of a fertilized ovum each month, and then be able to undergo constant change as the fetus grows in size. If fertilization of the ovum does not take place, it must repeat its cycle and await another opportunity. It is probably because of these complex anatomical changes the uterus must undergo that it is so fraught with medical and surgical problems.

The uterus is a hollow, pear-shaped, muscular pouch that is closed on the top end, the fundus, and open to the vagina via the cervix on the other. The fallopian tubes are attached to the sides of the upper part of the uterus and communicate with it. The far ends of the fallopian tubes (fimbria) sit above the ovaries, where they pick up the ovum. Besides producing the ovum, the ovaries produce hormones that increase the blood supply to the lining of the uterus. This causes a pro-

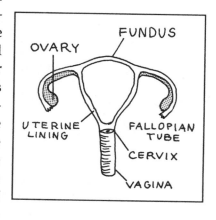

liferation and thickening of the uterine lining in preparation for implantation of a fertilized ovum. If implantation does not take place, the blood supply is severely reduced. Without adequate blood supply to nourish it, the uterine lining dies. This sloughing of the dead lining and subsequent bleeding is what we call menstruation.

Menstruation is not the function of the uterus, but a by-product of the reproductive process. If fertilization takes place, the embryo attaches to the lining, producing a placenta. The placenta then produces hormones of its own, which maintain the integrity of the uterine lining and the viability of the embryo. The uterus has the ability to enlarge from a pear-sized organ to one the size of a basketball, and then after delivery shrink to pear size again.

Fertilization does not take place in the uterus, as many people believe, but rather in the fallopian tubes. The fertilized ovum then migrates through the fallopian tube into the uterus, where it attaches to the uterine wall. Sometimes the

> It is probably because of the complex anatomical changes the uterus must undergo that it is so fraught with medical and surgical problems.

fertilized ovum becomes caught in the fallopian tube and does not reach the uterus. If the ovum continues to grow in the fallopian tube (ectopic pregnancy), it will eventually cause the fallopian tube to rupture. This is a true medical emergency and demands immediate surgical intervention to stop the profuse bleeding that can occur. I have personally been involved in many cases where the patient is rushed to surgery in shock from a ruptured ectopic pregnancy. The saving grace is that most of these patients are young, otherwise healthy women who can tolerate a short period of shock without residual effects.

Uterine cancer is the most common malignancy found in the female pelvis. Although uterine fibroids are more common in menstruating women, uterine cancer is more common in postmenopausal years. Vaginal bleeding in postmenopausal women is therefore of great concern because it could be a symptom of uterine cancer. Performing a D&C (dilatation and curettage) is both therapeutic and diagnostic in most noncancerous cases. The removed tissue can be examined under the microscope for a diagnosis and the uterine lining returned to a normal, nonprolific state. Hysterectomy (removal of the uterus), alone or in combination with radiation, is the treatment for uterine cancer.

Aftereffects

A common misconception is that the term *total hysterectomy* means also removing the fallopian tubes and ovaries. It does not. It means total removal of the uterus including the cervix. The fallopian tubes and ovaries are frequently removed (salpingo-oophorectomy) in older women at the time of hysterectomy or when surgery is performed for uterine cancer. If the ovaries are removed while a patient is still in the reproductive years, surgical menopause is produced. This is not because the patient no longer menstruates, but because of the loss of the ovarian hormones. Many authorities believe harmful side effects can develop without these hormones. Loss of calcium from bones and mood and body contour changes are a few of them. Most of the gynecologists I know prescribe hormones to counteract these problems for postmenopausal women unless contraindicated by cancer.

One-third of all women in this country will have a hysterectomy by age 65.

Symptoms

Hysterectomy is the most commonly performed abdominal surgery on women, and a high percentage of these are for fibroid tumors. These are benign tumors of smooth muscles that develop from the uterus. They grow during the reproductive years and decrease in size after menopause. These can be on the outside of the uterus projecting into the abdomen or on the inside of the uterine wall. They can be as small as a pea or as large as a volleyball. Most fibroid tumors don't cause any symptoms and are frequently only an incidental finding on a routine pelvic examination. Some, however, can cause a wide variety of symptoms. The most common is uterine bleeding, which occurs when they are in the lining of the uterine wall. This can be very resistant to treatment short of hysterectomy. The mere size of the fibroid can cause symptoms by pressing on other organs. A common example would be pressure on the bladder causing urinary frequency (the need to urinate often). They can also cause pain, infertility, discomfort during intercourse or spontaneous abortion.

It is a common occurrence for women to have abnormal uterine bleeding. In young women it could be from a miscarriage, when some of the products of conception are retained in the uterus. Or it could be that the monthly cycle of build up and sloughing of the uterine wall is disrupted. This can lead to abnormally long or heavy menstrual flows, with the causes running the gamut from hormone imbalance to emotional trauma. Some women have abnormal uterine bleeding requiring numerous D&Cs which only control the bleeding for a short time. This excessive blood loss causes anemia (not enough red blood cells) or painful abdominal cramping. Since it is the red blood cells that carry oxygen, anemia results in a substantial loss of energy. It is like trying to race a boat with only half the sails up. When anemia is due to this type of chronic blood loss, it responds well to iron pills once the problem is corrected.

Abnormal uterine bleeding, pain, or an abdominal mass are some of the more common gynecological symptoms that cause women to seek medical treatment. As discussed previously, there are many causes for these symptoms, and some

> The uterus has the ability to enlarge from a pear-sized organ to one the size of a basketball, and then after delivery shrink to pear size again.

require a hysterectomy to correct. A careful history and physical examination are of great value in helping to determine if symptoms require medical or surgical treatment.

Nonsurgical Treatment

Abnormal uterine bleeding, when caused by an imbalance of hormones, can be controlled with medications in most cases.

Uterine fibroids can often be watched if not causing symptoms because of their low incidence of malignancy. Periodic examinations are made to determine if they have undergone any change in size. Rapid increase in size may be a warning sign of malignant change. If bleeding is caused from a fibroid and the patient is near menopausal age, the bleeding will frequently stop with the onset of menopause.

SURGICAL PROCEDURES
D&C

Before having a hysterectomy many women undergo a D&C to try and correct their problem or to help make a diagnosis. To perform this surgery the opening of the uterus (the cervix) is dilated by inserting metal rods of increasing size through the vagina and into the cervical opening. This causes the cervical canal to stretch until it is large enough to allow an instrument with a sharp scoop on the end (a curette) to be passed through it. The inside of the uterus is then scraped with the curette, removing some of the lining. This is a relatively simple, safe surgery and is commonly done on an outpatient basis.

Vaginal Hysterectomy

The uterus can be surgically removed by an incision in the abdomen or from below by an incision in the vagina. The vaginal approach can't be used on women who have adhesions within the pelvis from prior surgeries or infections or those with a large uterus. As visibility is limited with this incision, it would be impossible to free up all the tissues and control bleeding. But for those who are a candidate for this approach, it offers a shorter and more comfortable postoperative recovery.

Delivering children through the vaginal canal causes damage to the supporting tissues of the urinary bladder and the rectum. This can cause urinary incontinence (leakage of urine) and constipation. Also the vagina can be stretched to the point of reducing sexual satisfaction for both partners. During a vaginal hysterectomy is a convenient time to have corrective surgery performed on these problems.

In vaginal hysterectomy the patient is given an anesthetic and her legs placed in stirrups. The surgical area is washed off with an antiseptic solution and a speculum is placed in the vagina. A catheter is inserted in the urinary bladder and the urine drained from it. This collapses the bladder, allowing for better visualization, and protects it from accidental injury during surgery. An incision is made at the back of the vagina, around the cervix, freeing it up from the vagina. Retractors are placed inside the incision allowing the surgeon to locate and surgically free up the uterus.

If the fallopian tubes are not going to be removed, they are freed from the sides of the uterus. If the fallopian tubes and ovaries are to be removed, the blood supply to them is tied off and cut. Very careful attention is given to any bleeding, which is promptly controlled. With the uterus removed, the end of the vagina which once held the cervix is now open and must be sutured closed. Any repair work on the supporting tissues of the bladder or rectum, if needed, can be conveniently done at this time.

Abdominal Hysterectomy

There are typically two types of incisions for abdominal hysterectomies, midline or a low transverse incision. The midline incision is just that, a vertical incision running down from just below the belly button to just above the pubic hairline. To my way of thinking this is an old-fashioned incision as it is cosmetically unsightly. The low transverse is made horizontally across the lower abdomen, just above the pubic hairline, and is invisible in any two-piece bathing suit I'd let my daughter wear. It is technically more difficult to operate through but worth it, as it tends to heal with less chance of developing a postoperative incisional hernia. Certainly there are special circumstances where a midline incision is more practical, as when a large tumor or dense adhesions are present.

As in the vaginal approach, the urinary bladder is emptied by catheterization to avoid injury. Once inside the abdominal cavity, the intestines are pushed out of the way into the upper abdomen. This is done with small cloth towels called sponges and metal retractors. The uterine fundus (top part) is held securely with a clamp. The fallopian tubes are severed from the sides of the uterus where they attach. The surgeon continues to dissect down the sides of the uterus, until the cervix is freed from the top of the vagina. Once free the uterus can be removed. This leaves the cut end of the vagina open to the abdominal cavity. This open end is sutured shut, possibly leaving the vagina shorter than before surgery. If the fallopian tubes and ovaries are to be removed, their blood supply and supporting tissues are freed from the pelvis. The uterus, fallopian tubes and ovaries can then be removed as one specimen. The surgeon then works his way up through the various layers, closing them in order. Finally the skin is closed and a dressing put over the incision. All tissue removed from the patient is sent to the laboratory for examination by a pathologist.

BREAST IMPLANTS

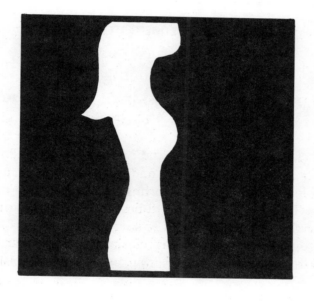

The breast is made up of tissues that don't have the ability to regain their shape after being stretched, making them very susceptible to the constant stress of gravity.

Description

We seem to have two different standards in our beauty-oriented society when it comes to female breast size. The female sex symbol in movies and magazine centerfolds is typically large bosomed. We all know of movie stars whose trademark is their greater-than-average bust size. Many of these Hollywood entertainers owe their large breasts not to their genes but to their plastic surgeons. On the other hand, the ideal fashion model is slender and small busted. Whatever their motivation, many 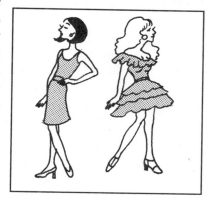 women are having breast implant surgery. The saying "Beauty is in the eye of the beholder" is certainly true in the area of the female breast.

There are other less controversial reasons for breast augmentation (enlargement). Some girls' breasts fail to develop during adolescence, leaving them with small, infantile breasts as women. Others are self-conscious about an inequality of breast size caused by developmental abnormality, injury or previous deforming surgery.

Some women with a very strong family history of breast cancer, after having several breast biopsies, elect to have the tissue in their breasts prophylactically (preventively) removed. They then have breast implantation surgery to regain their figure. With the implant lying *under* whatever breast tissue remains, an accurate breast examination can still be performed. Women, particularly young ones, who have had a mastectomy (surgical removal of the breast) sometimes want to have reconstructive breast surgery. Here the implant is invaluable in helping to shape the new breast.

The breast is made up of tissues that don't have the ability to regain their shape after being stretched, making them very susceptible to the constant stress of gravity. Over time these supporting tissues can break down, causing the breasts to become pendulous and lose their shape. Some breast implant surgery is done to return sagging, shapeless breasts to their original shape or, as one plastic surgeon says, "better than nature made them." If gravity can make people's eyelids sag, think what an effect it can have on the much larger breast. This is why I always advise women to wear a good supportive bra—gravity is always at work, so let's try to defeat it with good support. Unfortunately, as is common with so many other degenerative conditions, once the damage is done it is permanent.

Too Much of a Good Thing

At the other end of the spectrum are women with very large, heavy breasts, causing back and shoulder problems and making it hard to buy clothes that fit properly. Some large-breasted women, for these and other reasons, have surgery to reduce their breast size.

By a complicated surgical method of resecting sections out of the breast and suturing the opposite edges together, the size of the breast can be reduced. The nipple is, however, no longer in the appropriate position on the breast, making it necessary to cut the nipple and areola (colored area around the nipple) completely off the breast. Calculating where the nipple should now be located, the surgeon excises a circular area of skin from the breast at that point. He then sews the nipple and areola into this new location.

Reimplanting the nipple and areola in their new location

is, in effect, a skin graft. As with all skin grafts, there is always the possibility that the blood supply will not be adequate and the graft will die. If this happens, the plastic surgeon must perform another surgery to construct a new nipple out of tissue from another part of the body.

Misconceptions

There have been many nonsurgical approaches to breast enlargement. One was rubbing an irritating cream or ointment like cocoa butter on the breast, causing irritation and redness. It was thought that the increased redness was a sign of new blood vessels in the breast, which would cause breast-tissue proliferation and an increase in breast size. Actually, the blood vessels already present in the skin only dilated (increased in size), causing the reddened appearance. So, unfortunately, the only result was red, sore breasts of unchanged size.

Next came the female hormone craze, which did in some cases achieve breast enlargement. There were, however, many undesirable side effects, such as abnormal uterine bleeding, and only a small percentage of women were helped. The advent of the birth control pill brought a new dimension to hormone therapy and the first real medical success. But this still left many women who, for one reason or another, couldn't, shouldn't or wouldn't take the pill. And many women on the pill got less than the results they desired.

The breast is made up of a mixture of breast and fatty tissue, held in its classical shape by fibrous, supportive connective tissue. Because it has no muscle tissue, exercises to enlarge the breast are of no value. You can build up the chest wall muscles underlying the breast, thereby pushing the breasts forward. This might make the breasts appear larger than they actually are.

Next came silicone injections directly into the breast tissue. Silicone seemed like an ideal substance as it was resistant to breakdown by water—breast tissue is mostly water—and nonreactive to human tissues. This procedure was relatively painless, simple and at first seemed to offer good results. However, with the passage of time this technique came into disrepute as the silicone tended to clump, forming lumpy and unsightly breasts. It was also impossible to tell which lumps were silicone and which were tumors that needed to be removed, making breast examinations and subsequent evaluation very difficult. And once the silicon was injected, it was almost impossible to remove.

Finally came breast implants which, while plagued with problems early on, are quite successful today.

Surgical Procedure

It takes three to four hours to surgically insert breast implants. It can be done in a plastic surgeon's office with a local anesthetic and sedation or in a hospital or outpatient surgery center using a general anesthetic. The surgeon makes an incision below the breast and dissects *under* the breast tissue, forming a pocket below the existing breast tissue. Because a foreign body (the breast implant) is being inserted into this pocket, all bleeding must be stopped, as this could act as a focus for bacteria and lead to infection. Next the breast implant—a plastic bag filled with a gelatinous material—is fitted into the pocket.

The plastic surgeon has already discussed with the patient before surgery how large she would like her breasts to be. The size of the breast implant bags vary according to the size of the breasts requested—the larger the breast size, the larger the implant. But on average they are about the size of a child's bean bag.

The surgeon sutures closed the skin incision, taking care not to pierce the implant with a needle while sewing. Yes, I have seen implants punctured at the end of surgery, requiring removal and replacement—a very embarrassing moment for the plastic surgeon. Then he performs the same procedure on the other breast, making sure that both sides are

> The size of the breast implant bags vary...but on average they are about the size of a child's bean bag.

equal, not only in size, but also in symmetry. It is not always an easy matter to get both breasts to match and to be at the same level when standing. To me the miracle is that, even though the implants are relatively flat, the breasts assume a conical shape after their insertion. The resulting scar is in the natural crease under the breast and is usually hardly noticeable.

The early implants had a tendency over time to become hard and lose their natural appearance and fleshy feel. The newer implants have largely corrected this problem. However, in some women the body tries to wall off this foreign body by producing a fibrinous capsule around the implant. This becomes hard and painful, sometimes necessitating replacement of the implant.

Complications

There is no medical significance to small or pendulous breasts; the motivation for this type of surgery is cosmetic. For this reason most medical insurance companies will not

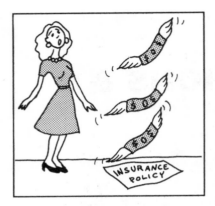

cover the cost of breast implant surgery. In addition to the monetary costs, there can be complications that take a mental and physical toll. As mentioned previously, the insertion of a foreign body (the implant) into the breast can lead to infection. Or, the breast implant can migrate out of its original location, up or down as well as sideways across the chest. The skin can even erode until the implant becomes exposed. Or it may become very hard and painful or collect pockets of fluid around it. I know of one young lady who, because of some of these complications, has had her breast implants replaced four times. For the majority of women, however, the results are satisfactory and the complications few.

QUESTIONS & ANSWERS

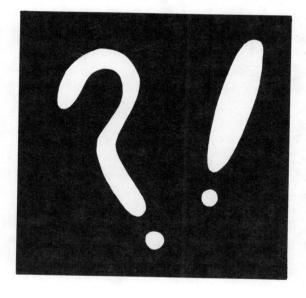

QUESTION: Is catgut suture really made from the intestines of cats?

ANSWER: Through the years many different materials have been used for sutures, ranging from horse and camel hair to gold and silver wires. Suture material can be divided into nonpermanent (absorbable) and permanent (nonabsorbable). The surgeon will choose the type of suture that best fits the needs of the specific circumstance at hand. For example, he will use an absorbable suture in an infected area so that it will disappear before it can act as a focus for infection. Oh yes, you can relax—catgut is an absorbable suture made from the intestines of sheep or cattle, not cats.

QUESTION: Why can't I drive home after outpatient surgery?

ANSWER: If surgery is performed with a local anesthetic and no sedation is given, the patient is usually allowed to drive himself home. If a patient is given any type of sedation or general anesthesia, however, he is not allowed to drive himself home. This is because these medications, without the patient being aware of it, impair judgment, reflexes and perception; he would be endangering himself and others if allowed to operate a motor vehicle too soon after sedation.

QUESTION: How do you find a good surgeon?

ANSWER: There is no easy answer to this question. I feel that the people who really know how good a surgeon is are the personnel in the operating room. So if you know an operating room nurse, technician or anesthesiologist, they would be a good referral source. Most people, however, do not know anyone in these categories. While not as good as operating room personnel, in my opinion, your own family doctor should be able to recommend a qualified surgeon. Most states have a medical board that will tell you if a surgeon has had any disciplinary action taken against him. Some will also inform you of any malpractice lawsuits settled against a doctor. (For a list of the states having medical boards, with their addresses and telephone numbers, see p. 144.) Also, check to see if a surgeon is certified by his specialty board; this will at least tell you that he has completed an approved training program. In my experience recommendations from nonmedical friends do not ensure getting the kind of expertise you are looking for as they are usually based on the surgeon's personality rather than his surgical ability.

QUESTION: What is a PCA pump?

ANSWER: The traditional method of administering pain-relieving postoperative narcotics has been by intramuscular (into the muscle) injection every three to four hours. The problems with this technique are (1) the patient must call and wait for the nurse to come, check the chart, load the syringe and finally give the shot, (2) it is given into the muscles where its slow absorption into the blood stream causes further delay in pain relief, and (3) the injection is painful.

The PCA (Patient Controlled Analgesia) pump is a machine containing the narcotic prescribed by the surgeon and connected to the patient by an intravenous line. The patient is given a control button that will administer a predetermined dose of the narcotic at the patient's discretion. There is a built-in time limit to how often the patient can self-administer the medication; with the frequency and dose limited by the settings of the PCA pump, the patient can't administer more than the maximum amount prescribed. The advantages of this method are (1) there is no delay in the administration of the medication so long as it is within the proper time frame, (2) the narcotic is administered into the blood stream with rapid onset of effects, (3) because it goes directly into the blood stream only a small dose is required, (4) since only a small dose is required it can be repeated at frequent intervals, and (5) the patient feels that he is in control. Because of these factors patients usually use a smaller total dose of narcotic with the PCA pump than with the older intramuscular method.

QUESTION: Why do surgeons leave drains in after surgery?

ANSWER: The surgeon attempts to stop bleeding as much as possible during surgery so that the the operative site will be as dry as possible when he closes up the wound. In some cases it is impossible to stop all the oozing of blood from certain areas. This oozing is not of a magnitude that will affect the patient's general condition, but will accumulate locally in the operative site. This collection of blood retards healing and increases the incidence of infection. A drain is usually a flat, ribbon-shaped length of rubber, but can even be a piece of plastic tubing with suction on the end. The purpose of the drain is to allow any fluid that might accumulate to flow out around the drain onto a dressing or into a container. Anywhere from one to seven days after surgery the drain is removed by gently pulling it out.

QUESTION: What is an autologous blood transfusion?

ANSWER: With many surgeries a high probability exists that there will be a need to replace blood lost during the procedure. If this is an elective surgery, the patient can have the blood bank collect several units of his own blood over a two-week period just prior to surgery. This blood can then be given back to the patient during surgery without fear of hepatitis, AIDS or incompatible blood reaction.

QUESTION: As surgeons wear gloves during surgery, why do they scrub their hands prior to surgery?

ANSWER: The traditional five-minute hand scrub prior to gloving is necessary for several reasons. The thin gloves worn by the surgeons often tear, exposing the surgeon's skin. A surgical needle could inadvertently puncture the glove, contaminating the needle and possibly the wound. Also there could be tiny, unnoticed holes in the gloves which could allow any bacteria on the surgeon's hands to pass into the surgical field. This has become even more apparent with the closer examination of protective rubber goods since the onset of AIDS.

QUESTION: What is the difference between an anesthesiologist and an anesthetist?

ANSWER: An anesthesiologist is a medical doctor who has taken two to three years of additional training in the speciality of anesthesiology. A nurse anesthetist is a nurse who has taken specialized training in anesthesia.

QUESTION: Why do they put a grounding pad on the patient at the start of surgery?

ANSWER: One of the most frequently used methods to stop bleeding of small blood vessels during surgery is with electrical cautery. This is a pencil-shaped probe with a metal tip that is held next to a bleeding blood vessel. At the push of a button the electrical current burns the end of the blood vessel, coagulating the blood and sealing off the blood vessel. The grounding pad is necessary to complete the electrical circuit. The grounding pad dissipates the electrical current over a large area; without it any portion of the body could act as a ground. If this should be a small area, the electrical current passing through could cause the skin and underlying tissues to heat up and an electrical burn could result.

QUESTION: Why can't I have a spinal anesthetic for breast surgery?

ANSWER: Besides causing numbness of the skin and underlying tissues, spinal anesthetics also cause paralysis of muscles. Roughly speaking, the area of muscle paralysis parallels the area of numbness. This level of numbness can be raised or lowered by several factors controlled by the anesthesiologist. If a spinal anesthetic were administered at a high enough level to numb the skin of the breasts, it would also paralyze the diaphragm and chest muscles—the muscles of respiration—and with them paralyzed the patient would be unable to breathe. This is why spinal anesthesia is usually not given if the area to be operated on is above the level of the belly button.

QUESTION: Why do some people develop keloids in their surgical incision?

ANSWER: A keloid is a thick, raised, unsightly, tender scar that can form in the surgical incision. It seems to be an exaggerated response of the healing process. The cause is unknown, but is more common in dark-skinned people and over areas where there is increased skin tension such as the breastbone (sternum). Other common areas are ears, chin, neck and shoulders. As simple a thing as piercing the ears to wear earrings could cause unsightly keloids to form on the earlobes. Once formed they can be treated with x-rays, cryotherapy (freezing temperatures) or corticosteroid injections. When simply excised, they tend to recur if not treated by one of the above modalities.

QUESTION: Why can't I see the patient in the recovery room?

ANSWER: Because a patient emerging from an anesthetic requires very close observation. There is a high ratio of nurses to patients in the recovery room; concerned family members or friends tend to obstruct the smooth flow of patient care. Also they do not understand the different states of awareness and disorientation that can be experienced on awakening by some patients and distract the nurses with questions.

QUESTION: If they find a lump in my breast with a mammogram (x-ray of the breast) that the doctor can't feel, how is he going to find it during surgery?

ANSWER: It is not uncommon for a lump to be found on a mammogram that can't be felt by the surgeon. It is located at surgery with the aid of a radiologist and the x-ray department. A radiologist inserts several long, thin needles into the breast, aiming where he thinks the lump is with the mammogram as a guide. As these are very fine needles, no anesthetic is required. If by repeat x-rays the needles are not found to be in the lump, he withdraws and redirects them as indicated by the x-rays. This process is repeated until the needle is in the lump. The patient now goes to the operating room and is put under anesthesia. The surgeon follows the needles down to the lump and excises it. The lump can be sent back to the radiologist and x-rayed to confirm that it matches the lump previously seen.

SECRETARIES OF STATE MEDICAL EXAMINING BOARDS

ALABAMA STATE BOARD OF MEDICAL EXAMINERS
P. O. Box 946
Montgomery, AL 36102-0946
(205) 832-6890

ALASKA BOARD OF MEDICAL EXAMINERS
Division of Occupational Licensing
Pouch D, Juneau, AK 99811
(907) 465-2541

ARIZONA STATE BOARD OF MEDICAL EXAMINERS
5060 N. 19th Avenue, #300
Phoenix, AZ 85015
(602) 255-3751

ARIZONA BOARD OF OSTEOPATHIC EXAMINERS IN MEDICINE & SURGERY
2020 W. Indian School Road, Suite 46, Phoenix, AZ 85015
(602) 265-5073

ARKANSAS STATE MEDICAL BOARD
P. O. Box 102
Harrisburg, AR 72432
(501) 578-2677

CALIFORNIA BOARD OF MEDICAL QUALITY ASSURANCE
1430 Howe Avenue
Sacramento, CA 95825
(916) 920-6393

CALIFORNIA BOARD OF OSTEOPATHIC EXAMINERS
921 11th Street, #1201
Sacramento, CA 95314
(916) 322-4306

COLORADO BOARD OF MEDICAL EXAMINERS
132 State Services Building
Denver, CO 80203
(303) 866-2468

CONNECTICUT MEDICAL EXAMINING BOARD
79 Elm Street, Hartford, CT 06106
(203) 566-3033

DELAWARE BOARD OF MEDICAL PRACTICE
Margaret O'Neill Building, 3rd Floor/P. O. Box 1401
Dover, DE 19901
(302) 736- 4753

DISTRICT OF COLUMBIA COMMISSION ON LICENSURE TO PRACTICE THE HEALING ARTS
605 G Street, NW, Room 202, Lower Level
Washington, DC 20001
(202) 727-5365

FLORIDA BOARD OF MEDICAL EXAMINERS
130 N. Monroe Street
Tallahassee, FL 32301
(904) 488-0595

FLORIDA BOARD OF OSTEOPATHIC MEDICAL EXAMINERS
130 N. Monroe Street
Tallahasse, FL 32301
(904) 488-0595

GEORGIA COMPOSITE BOARD OF MEDICAL EXAMINERS
166 Pryor Street, SW
Atlanta, GA 30303
(404) 656-7067

HAWAII BOARD OF MEDICAL
EXAMINERS
P. O. Box 541, Honolulu, HI 96809
(808) 548-6245

IDAHO STATE BOARD OF
MEDICINE
700 W. State Street, Boise ID 83729
(208) 334-2822

ILLINOIS DEPARTMENT OF
REGISTRATION & EDUCATION
320 W. Washington Street
Springfield, IL 62786
(217) 785-0820

INDIANA HEALTH
PROFESSIONS SERVICE
BUREAU
1 American Square, Suite 1020
Indianapolis, IN 46282
(317) 232-2960

IOWA STATE BOARD OF
MEDICAL EXAMINERS
State Capital Complex
Des Moines, IA 50319
(515) 281-5171

KANSAS STATE BOARD OF
HEALING ARTS
900 SW Jackson, Suite 553
Topeka, KS 66612
(913) 296-7413

KENTUCKY STATE BOARD OF
MEDICAL LICENSURE
3532 Ephraim McDowell Drive
Louisville, KY 40205
(502) 456-2220

LOUISIANA STATE BOARD OF
MEDICAL EXAMINERS
830 Union Street, #100
New Orleans, LA 70112
(504) 524-6763

MAINE STATE BOARD OF
REGISTRATION IN MEDICINE
RFD #3, Box 461
Waterville, ME 04901
(207) 873-2184

MARYLAND BOARD OF
MEDICAL EXAMINERS
201 W. Preston Street, 5th Floor
Baltimore, MD 21201
(301) 383-2020

MASSACHUSETTS BOARD OF
REGISTRATION IN MEDICINE
Leverett Saltonstall Building
100 Cambridge Street, Room 1507
Boston, MA 02202
(617) 727-3086

MICHIGAN BOARD OF
MEDICINE
P. O. Box 30018
Lansing, MI 48908
(517) 373-0680

MICHIGAN BOARD OF
OSTEOPATHIC MEDICINE &
SURGERY
905 Southland, Lansing, MI 43909
(517) 373-1655

MINNESOTA STATE BOARD
OF MEDICAL EXAMINERS
717 Delaware Street, SE, Suite 352
Minneapolis, MN 55414
(612) 623-5534

MISSISSIPPI STATE BOARD OF
MEDICAL LICENSURE
P. O. Box 1700, Jackson, MS 39205
(601) 354-6645

MISSOURI STATE BOARD OF
REGISTRATION FOR THE
HEALING ARTS
P. O. Box 4
Jefferson City, MO 65102
(314) 751-2334

MONTANA STATE BOARD OF
MEDICAL EXAMINERS
1424 Ninth Avenue
Helena, MT 59620
(406) 449-3737

NEBRASKA BOARD OF
EXAMINERS IN MEDICINE &
SURGERY
P. O. Box 95007, Lincoln, NE 68509
(402) 471-2115

NEVADA STATE BOARD OF
MEDICAL EXAMINERS
P. O. Box 7238, Reno, NV 89510
(702) 329-2559

NEW HAMPSHIRE BOARD OF
REGISTRATION IN MEDICINE
Health & Welfare Building
Hazen Drive, Concord, NH 03301
(603) 271-4501

NEW JERSEY STATE BOARD OF
MEDICAL EXAMINERS
28 West State Street, Room 914
Trenton, NJ 08608
(609) 292-4843

NEW MEXICO STATE BOARD
OF MEDICAL EXAMINERS
227 E. Palace Avenue, Suite O
Santa Fe, NM 87501
(505) 827-2215

NEW MEXICO BOARD OF
OSTEOPATHIC MEDICAL
EXAMINERS
718 Lomas Blvd., NW
Albuquerque, NM 87102
(505) 247-0541

NEW YORK BOARD FOR
MEDICINE
Cultural Educational Center
Room 3029, Empire State Plaza
Albany, NY 12230
(518) 474-3830

NORTH CAROLINA STATE
BOARD OF MEDICAL
EXAMINERS
Suite 214, 222 N. Person Street
Raleigh, NC 27601
(919) 833-5321

NORTH DAKOTA STATE
BOARD OF MEDICAL
EXAMINERS
City Center Plaza
418 E. Broadway, Suite C-10
Bismarck, ND 58501
(701) 223-9485

OHIO STATE MEDICAL BOARD
65 S. Front Street, #510
Columbus, OH 43215
(614) 466-3934

OKLAHOMA BOARD OF
MEDICAL EXAMINERS
P. O. Box 18256
Oklahoma City, OK 73154
(405) 848-6841

OREGON BOARD OF MEDICAL
EXAMINERS
317 Alder Street, 1002 Loyalty
Building, Portland, OR 97204
(503) 229-5770

PENNSYLVANIA STATE
BOARD OF MEDICAL
EDUCATION & LICENSURE
P. O. Box 2649
Harrisburg, PA 17105-2646
(717) 787-2381

PENNSYLVANIA STATE
BOARD OF OSTEOPATHIC
MEDICAL EXAMINERS
P. O. Box 2649
Harrisburg, PA 17105
(717) 787-8504

PUERTO RICO BOARD OF
MEDICAL EXAMINERS
Program of Quality Control of
Health Services
Box 9342, Santurce, PR 00908
(809) 722-2028

RHODE ISLAND BOARD OF
MEDICAL REVIEW
100 India Street
Providence, RI 02903
(401) 277-3855

SOUTH CAROLINA STATE
BOARD OF MEDICAL
EXAMINERS
1315 Blanding Street
Columbia, SC 29201
(803) 758-3361

SOUTH DAKOTA STATE
BOARD OF MEDICAL &
OSTEOPATHIC EXAMINERS
608 West Avenue North
Sioux Falls, SD 57104
(605) 336-1965

TENNESSEE STATE BOARD OF
MEDICAL EXAMINERS
320 R. S. Gass State Office Building
Ben Allen Road
Nashville, TN 37216
(615) 741-7280

TENNESSEE STATE BOARD OF
OSTEOPATHIC EXAMINERS
320 R. S. Gass State Office Building
Ben Allen Road
Nashville, TN 37216
(615) 741-7280

TEXAS STATE BOARD OF
MEDICAL EXAMINERS
P. O. Box 13562, Capitol Station
Austin, TX 78711
(512) 452-1078

UTAH DIVISION OF
REGISTRATION
160 E. 300 S./P. O. Box 5802
Salt Lake City, UT 84110
(801) 530-6628

VERMONT BOARD OF
MEDICAL PRACTICE
109 State Street
Montpelier, VT 05602
(802) 828-2363

VIRGINIA STATE BOARD OF
MEDICINE
517 W. Grace Street/P. O. Box
27708, Richmond, VA 23261
(804) 786-0575

WASHINGTON DEPARTMENT
OF LICENSING
P. O. Box 9649, Olympia, WA 98504
(206) 753- 1369

WASHINGTON BOARD OF
OSTEOPATHIC MEDICINE &
SURGERY
P. O. Box 9649, Olympia, WA 98504
(206) 753-2205

WEST VIRGINIA BOARD OF
MEDICINE
3412 Chesterfield Avenue, SE
Charleston, WV 25304
(304) 925-4061

WISCONSIN MEDICAL
EXAMINING BOARD
1400 E. Washington Avenue
Madison, WI 53702
(608) 266-2811

WYOMING BOARD OF
MEDICAL EXAMINERS
Hathaway Building, 4th Floor
Cheyenne, WY 82002
(307) 777-7121 or 777-7122

Index